PUBLIC HEALTH AND SOCIAL ASPECTS

PUBLIC HEALTH AND SOCIAL ASPECTS

By

PROF. (COL.) P.K. DUTTA

KHAMA PUBLISHERS
NEW DELHI

PUBLIC HEALTH AND SOCIAL ASPECTS

First Published in India 1998

ISBN 81-85495-48-3

Published by:
A. Banerjee
for Khama Publishers
1770, Khawaspura, Pataudi House
Daryaganj, New Delhi-110002

Laser typeset at:
Printline
12-H, New Daryaganj Road,
New Delhi-110002

Printed at:
Super Printers
1893, Gali Behrem Beg,
Lal Kuan, Delhi

Dedicated
To
My Parents

Contents

SECTION IV
HEALTH EDUCATION

SECTION V
MISCELLANEOUS

Preface

Most of today's health problems are attributed to biological, social, environmental and individual factors for causation of illness and also for the subsequent progress in natural history of the disease. There is no denial of the fact that the social environment is very important in relation to health and disease of the human population.

With growing industrialisation, urbanisation and control of communicable diseases specially of parasitic and bacterial origin, there is emergence of non-communicable disease. In today's world, effects of social environment has distinct impact on the morbidity pattern specially in rural areas and urban slums. Many of the important public health problems are also related to life styles of people belonging to different strata of the societies and examples are many – Diabetes, obesity, coronary heart disease, Alcohal and drug abuses. The changes in value system also are reflected in an increasing trend of diseases associated with modern world.

The effects of social environemnt reflect on the complex of psycho social aspects influencing health and disease of the individauls, the communities and the nations. The social environment is unique to man and include cultural values, customs, habits, attitudes, beliefs, education, income, occupation, standard of community life and impact of social and political organisations. Hence it is essential to have proper understanding of social sciences in general and sociology and cultural antropology in particular in order to appreciate impact of social environment and it's adverse effects on health and diseases. Sociology is the behaviour of man in society. The man's behaviour is affected not only by biological and physical environemnt, but also by social environment.

It is now being gradually realised by researchers and scientists from various disciplines that a number of factors are associated with health and disease. Some of the behavioural sciences including sociology, anthropology and psychology are closely interrelated with natural history of many diseases - right from etiology, diagnosis, preventive measures and rehabilitation. A holistic and interdisciplinary approach, therefore, is essential for research workers drawn from different disciplines including health and social sciences. Not many social scientists and public health specialists either singularly or jointly have indertaken relevant research studies to corelate social aspects of disease and health. The author had conducted a number of studies during the last 3 decades of his professional career including knowledge, application and practice (KAP) studies in the fields of communicable disease, family planning and MCH care.

The author has experienced during 25 years in medical teaching and research, that not many empirical studies/relevant literature on the subject could be cited for training post graduate students in medicine. Even for undergraduate students, this is a definite 'felt need' of psycho-social studies in health and disease, which could be a source of inspiration for medical sociologists. The community based social sciences research in the field of community medicine is very few and far between. Keeping this in mind, the author decided to compile the relevant articles/studies that were undertaken either by him, his colleagues and post-graudate students, during his 5 years tenure at AFMC, Pune and subsequently.

The importance of health education has been realised immensely during last few years so much so that it has been recognised as a speciality. Few national institutions like All India Institute of Hygiene and Public Health, Calcutta, Central Health Education Bureau, New Delhi, Gandhigram Inst. of Rural Development, Madurai, had been conducting Post Gradurate Diploma courses on the subject i.e., Diploma in Health Education. The reason for attaching so much imporatnce to the subject was because educators/planners realised that utilisation of health care delivery system etc.

after elaborate planning, flop or remain fully under utilised because of lack of awareness among the beneficiaries. Hence it has been realised that clientele, for whom the health programme is meant, have to be properly educated and motivated, before rich dividends can be accrued. International Health agencies like WHO, UNICEF have been laying emphasis on the community participation and their full involment if we want to ensure optimal utilisation and active participation by the community. After gathering details on the health programme and after fully motivated only full participation by the community can be ensured.

This book is collection of 28 such articles which is divided into 6 sections.

Seciton 1 deals with medio social aspects of few communicable diseases, namely diarrhoeal diseases, sexually transmitted diseases, Measles and Smallpox. In this section, certain customs and beliefs among the study subjects about small pox and measles have also been studied.

Section 2 dealing with blindness has focussed on medicosocal and psychosocial profile of blind inmates of few homes.

Section 3 has highlighted about the medicosocial study of Menstrual Regulators (MR) & Medical Termination of Pregnancy (MTP) acceptors and also demographic profile of tubectomy acceptors.

Utilisation of health services by high risk children and of 'high risk' pregnant mothers have been brought out in Section 4 thus depicting causes of underutilisation of these essential services in slum areas.

In Section 4 a few articles on health education have been incorporated. These have been presented in a wider canvas and articles include smoking and its hazards, medicosocial problems of today's youth, geriatric population and their various problems, anaemia in pregnancy and cancer cervix, considered as scourge of women. This chapter also addresses other health and social issues like psychosocial aspects of hearing loss, diarrhoeal diseases under 5 children, population explosion and menace of intestinal helminthiasis.

Last chapter (Section 5) deals with a variety of other interesting topics life medicosocial study of paraplegics; tobacco smoking habits of army personnel, psychosocial profile of orphans, women to women education in devivery of non-formal health care, scope of Health System Research (HSR) in CSSM programme, India's preparation for disaster reduction and World Mental Health : Issues and Challenges.

In this book, an attempt has been made to present and analyse some of medicosocial and psychosocial issues related to health and disease.

The persons who initiated me in studying and writing articles on attitudes and beliefs about smallpox is none less than my revered teacher, Late Dr J. E. Park who has been one of the stalwarts in the field of community medicine. While I was enrolled as a postgraduate student in mid sixties under him, Dr. Park advised me to also initiate a research project on anthropological aspects of smallpox though my main topic of MD thesis was Evaluation of National Smallpox Eradication Pragramme in Gwalior District. The first article of my professional career on attitude and beliefs about smallpox was published in Armed Forces Medical Journal about 3 decades ago. Later on, I was granted 2 years study leave in late seventies and then I had the previlege of working with Prof. D. Banerjee at Jawaharlal Nehru Univeristy. He is also well known for his knowledge and command in the field of medical sociology and that too for his original and pioneering reserch. While working under him, I have also learnt a lot of various aspects of social sciences which could be applied in the field of social medicine. Both, Late Dr. J. Park and Dr. D. Banerjee my revered teachers inspired me to work in this field.

As mentioned earlier, very few studies have been conducted specially by the medical scientists in social aspects of health and disease. During the last two decades or so, though, few social scientists like Dr. K. Hasan, Dr. Sahu, Dr. Banerjee, etc. had undertaken a number of research studies which were mainly community based but hardly any medical scientists tried to initiate such projects. Even on review of literature, it was found that very few books/articles were available on this aspect. While teaching the undergraduate and postgraduate students at AFMC, Pune and most of the studies incorporated in the present publication is outcome of their research projects aundertaken by faculty members or postgraduate students. Few of my collegues were also keen to undertake projects on social aspects of health and were mostly community based projects. Prof. (Col.) A.C. Urmil, Dr. S.S. Ganguly and Late Col. (Dr.) T.K.G. Choudhary, my close friends and colleagues also had undertaken a number of studies based on social sciences. Other academic collegues and most of whom were postgraduate students during my tenure at AFMC whose names are worth mentiioning in bringing out the studies are Late Lt. Cols M. Kulkarni, Leo Vaz, Goutam Ghose, K.K. Sharma, P.K. Singh, Bhushan Kumar and S.K. Agarwal. All these colleagues from Army Medical Corps had been either jointly or singly working on various medico social aspects of health and disease. Col (Retd) Gopinathan, Prof. P.K. Somaya of, Karad Institute of Medical Sciences, Maharastra and Col. A.C. Urmil had always encourging me to take-up suitable research projects to correlate social sciences in health field. Inadvertantly, if any of my colleague's name has not been included, I owe an apology to them.

I would like to take this opportunity to thank Mr. Anupam Benerjee of Khama Publishers, Ansari Road, New Delhi and printers for bringing out the book in record time.

My thanks are also due to my wife Dr. (Mrs.) Mahuya Dutta and my children Pratik and Amrita for bearing with me while preparing the manuscript of the publication.

mainly community based but hardly any medical scientist tried to initiate such projects. Even on review of literature, it was found that very few books/articles were available on this aspect. While teaching the undergraduate and postgraduate students of AFMC, Pune and most of the studies incorporated in the present publication is outcome of their research projects undertaken by faculty members or postgraduate students. Few of my colleagues were also keen to undertake projects on social aspects of health and were mostly community based projects. Prof (Col) A.G. Urmil, Dr S.S. Ganguly and Late Col (Dr.) T.K.G. Choudhary, my close friends and colleagues also had undertaken a number of studies based on social sciences. Other academic colleagues and most of whom were postgraduate students during my tenure at AFMC whose names are worth mentioning in bringing out the studies are Late Lt. Cols M. Kulkarni, Lao Vas, Gautam Ghosh, N.K. Sharma, P.K. Singh, Ghoshan Kumar and S.K. Agarwal. All these colleagues from Army Medical Corps had been either jointly or singly working on various medico social aspects of health and disease. Col (Retd) Gopinath, Prof. P.K. Sohoni of Karad Institute of Medical Sciences, Maharashtra and Col A.G. Urmil had always encouraging me to take up social research projects to correlate social sciences in health field. Inadvertantly, if any of my colleague's name has not been included, I owe an apology to them.

I would like to take this opportunity to thank Mr. Anupam Banerjee of Khanna Publishers, Ansari Road, New Delhi and printers for bringing out the book in record time.

My thanks are also due to my wife Dr. (Mrs.) M. Bhatt Dutta and my children Pratik and Amrita for bearing with me while preparing the manuscript of the publication.

SECTION I

COMMUNICABLE DISEASES

Chapter–1

Knowledge, Attitude and Beliefs About Measles and Vaccination Coverage in a Rural Area

Asbstract

In the present study, an attempt was made to collect data on the attitude, belief and customs of mothers regarding occurrence of measles among children in a rural area in Jammu region. Their views on the various aspects of the disease have been highlighted in this article. Simultaneously an effort was also made to evaluate the measles vaccination coverage in the study area (UIP). This study brings out the scope of health education in the eventual goal of eradicating measles in the country.

Introduction

Measles is one of the common communicable diseases of the childhood and has been accorded priority by WHO specially in developing countries. This is because at every fifteen seconds a child dies from this disease in the world taking a toll of 2 million children every year (1). Virtually every unprotected child will contract the disease, which may be fatal for those who are already weakened by malnutrition (2). Complications occur in about thirty percent of cases and include otitis media, diarrhoea, blindness and encephalitis. In India, around 1,00,000 measles cases are reported every year with a case fatality rate of around 190 per 1, 00, 000 population. (3)

Part of the effort of achieving 85 percent immunisation against measles under Universal Immunization Programme (UIP) in our country by 1990 needs to be directed in mobilising the community, since their potential is enormous and their involvement is indispensable (4). Acceptability of the programme largely will depend on chanelising certain wrong ideas, attitudes and beliefs in the correct direction.

In view of the above, the present study was undertaken to ascertain the attitude, beliefs and customs regarding the occurrence, mode of transmission, complications of the disease as well as to determine the extent of vaccination coverage. The study could not be compared with other KAP studies on measles as no similar literature was encountered.

Material and Methods

The present study was undertaken for a period of two months i.e. January-March 1988 in two villages namely Rakh Muthi and Khour located about 43 and 48 kms respectively from Jammu city. The interview technique was adopted and relevant data was recorded in a pretested schedule. The study population consisted of 150 mothers of the two study villages. The families were selected from those mothers having children below 5 years of age. Simultaneously an attempt was also made to ascertain the immunisation coverage against measles among the children of the study population.

Results and Discussion

(i) Socio-Economic status : The percentage of families studied in relation to their socio-economic status is shown in Table 1 below.

Table 1
Distribution of families according to socio-economic status

Social Class	*No. of Families*	*Percen-tage*	*No. of Children below 5 years*	*Percentage*
I	–	–	–	–
II	30	20	47	17.2
III	40	26.66	73	26.7
IV	68	45.33	122	44.6
V	12	8.0	31	11.5
Total	150	100.00	273	100.0

The socio-economic status of family was determined as per the Kupuswamy scale. Most of families (72 percent) belonged to the III and IV group.

(ii) Knowledge about spread of the disease: It is very well known that people have divergent views about the spread of various communicable disease including measles. The opinion of the study subjects regarding mode of spread of the disease is shown in Table 2.

Table 2
Views of the respondents regarding spread of Measles

S. No.	*Mode of Spread*	*No. of persons responding*	*Percentage*
1.	Don't know	90	60.0
2.	Sneezing and coughing	24	16.0
3.	Bad air	23	15.3
4.	Bad food	11	7.3
5.	Unclean hands	5	3.3
6.	Bad weather	5	3.3
7.	Insects	4	2.6
8.	Any other method	3	2.0
	Total	166*	

* Few respondents gave more than one answer.

It is evident from Table 2 that majority of the mothers did not have correct knowledge about the spread of the disease. The facts that people had more than one view about the spread of measles indicated their ignorance about the disease transmission. Hence, there is scope for health education of lay people, especially mothers. Dissemination of correct information about spread of measles is an important step in containment of the disease.

(iii) Age at occurrence : Mothers were asked about their opinion regarding the age of occurrence of measles. Their responses are shown in Table 3.

Table 3
Distribution of mothers according to knowledge of age at occurrence

Age in years	*Numbers*	*Percentage*
Upto 12 months	0	-
2 - 4	120	80
5 - 14	20	13.3
15+	10	6.7
Total	150	100.0

Table 3 shows that 80 percent of the mothers interviewed mentioned that measles is a disease of childhood. In this regard most of the respondents were correct. On the contrary a few study subjects were of the opinion (6.66 percent) that the disease affected the people in adulthood.

It is interesting to note that the majority of the children of the respondents were found to have suffered from the disease between one to two years of their age.

(iv) Views on the seasonal incidence : Study subjects were also asked about their views on seasonal incidence of the disease. Almost three-fourth of the study subjects (73.33%) interviewed mentioned that the disease occurred mainly during summer months though

12.6 and 81 percent were of the opinion tht the disease was more prevalent during winter months and rainy season respectively. However, 6.0 percent of the interviewees expressed that the disease could occur in any season.

Based on scientific knowledge, it was found that the respondents were far from the truth since the disease is prevalent throughout the year with maximum cases and outbreaks occurring during winter month. (5)

(v) Views on complications of measles : All the interviewees were of the opinion of Measles (KHASRA) as a distinct disease entity. 49.82 percent of interviewees mentioned pneumonia as one of the complications.

(vi) Action on occurence of a case: When questioned on implementing the control measures following occurrence of a case in the family, 34 percent of the respondents said that they would consult a private practitioner whereas only 9.4 percent were in favour of admission to a hospital. 15.6 percent of the interviewees, however, did not feel the need to seek medical advice at all and only 10 percent of the mothers were in favour of isolation of the patient. Most of the people underestimated the importance of measles considering it to be a mild and routine childhood disease not requiring active intervention.

(vii) Type of diet which should be given to a child suffering from Measles (food prejudices): Respondents were asked about the diet which was best shited for a measles patient. Their replies are tabulated in Table 4.

Table 4 reveals that majority of mothers preferred to give liquid diet (63.3 percent) to the measles patients while 21.3 percent expressed about some restrictions e.g. no fried food or nothing hot and spicy should be given.

Table 4
Distribution of mothers as per their views on food prejudices

Sl. No.	*Type of Food*	*Numbers Responding*	*Percentage*
1.	Liquid	98	65.3
2.	Some specific restrictions	32	21.3
3.	Normal diet	11	7.3
4.	Semi solid Food	5	3.5
5.	Solid food	-	-
6.	Balanced diet	4	2.6
	Total	150	100.0

The immunisation coverage

Measles tends to be very severe among malnourished children and they are likely to be encountered more in the remote and rural settings. The disease in such cases carried a mortality 400 times higher than well nourished children. Restrictions on diet as considered necessary by mothers would only aggravate the chan~es of fatality in an already malnourished child.

Measles vaccine offers life long protection and since this had been introduced already, it was also decided to ascertain the immunisation coverage in the various age groups, which is shown in Table 5.

Table 5
Immunisatioin coverage according to age group

Sl. No.	*Age Group*	*Total No. of children in the age group*	*No. vaccinated*	*Percentage vaccinated*
1.	6 months to 1 year	48	21	43.7
2.	1 to 2 years	57	27	47.4
3.	2 to 3 years	45	07	15.5
4.	3 to 4 years	58	00	00.0
5.	4 to 5 years	65	00	00.0
	Total	273	55	20.1

It is quite apparent from the Table 5, that the percentage of children vaccinated was higher in the younger age group and progressively decreased with the increase in age. Though vaccine had been made available for last few years, but it is catching up fast with the beneficiaries in rural areas. Probably this may be attributed to better awareness among the lay people. Still is has to go a long way before achieving our desired goal of 85 percent immunisation of susceptible population by 1995.

It is obvious that there is wide scope of health education for mothers as disseminating knowledge about various aspects of the disease viz age at occurrence, mode of spread, seasonal incidence and diet for a child suffering from the disease are concerned. Though vaccination coverage was satisfactory considering the availability of vaccine, but sustained educational programme for beneficiaries is still indicated.

References

1. Universal Immunisation Programme (1988). Communicable Disease Bulletin, 5:2.
2. Morley David (1973). Paediatric Priorities in Developing world, Butterworth.
3. Park, J.E. (1987). Textbook of Preventive Medicine, p 123.
4. Comstock. G.W. (1975). American J. Epi 101-37.
5. Sehgal, S. (1988). Vaccination Coverage Survey. Communicable disease Bulletin, 5: 13-17.

Chapter-2

Medico-social Profile of Under Five Children Suffering From Diarrhoeal Diseases

Abstract

A total of 76 children under 5 years of age were studied for various diarrhoeal diseases. The study showed that the incidence of diarrhoea was more in lower socio-economic groups and was inversely proportional to the literacy status of mothers. Dehydration and fever were present in 78.95 and 75.00 per cent cases respectively, Majority of diarrhoeal cases were found to be suffering from malnutrition. 50 per cent mothers of the children had no knowledge about oral rehydration therapy (ORT), underlying the need for health education of mothers particularly regarding ORT.

Introduction

Almost two third of the 14 million child deaths each year are accounted for by just 4 specific causes - diarrhoea, respiratory infection, measles and neonatal tetanus. Out of these, the diarrhoeal diseases account for nearly 4 million deaths (28%). Approximately 60 per cent of these deaths are due to dehydration and therefore, largely preventable through oral rehydration therapy (ORT) (1).

In India, children under five years of age constitute 17 per cent of the population (2). On an average each child suffers 2 episodes of diarrhoea per year and out of these 1-4% of the episodes prove to be fatal. In developing countries the vicious cycle between diarrhoea and malnutrition, poor environmental sanitation, inadequate safe water supply, improper disposal of excreta, fly nuisance, overcrowding, ignorance and superstition have contributed to persistence of diarrhoeal disease in the community. A number of clinical and etiological studies on diarrhoea among children have been carried out, but only a few studies have dealt with the social, environmental and medical aspects comprehensively. The present study was therefore, undertaken to cover all these aspects of diarrhoeal diseases among children.

Material and Methods:

All 76 children under 5 years age, admitted in pediatric wards of Command Hospital (SC) Pune during the period of seven months in 1987, comprised the study subjects. A pretested and suitably modified schedule was used to record all relevant data on various medico social factors under study. This was followed by home visits to assess the socio-economic, cultural and environmental factors. Socio-economic status was worked out as per scale (urban) suggested by Kuppuswamy. Due to certain limitation in laboratory facilities, viral agents and pathogenic E-coil could not be serotyped.

Observations:

A total of 290 children under 5 years of age were admitted in the hospital during the period of study which included 186 male children (64.14%) and 104 female children (35.86%). A total number of 76 diarrhoeal cases comprised 26.20% of the total admissions and included 48 male children (63.16%) and 28 female children (36.84%).

Table I
Distribution of diarrhoeal cases by Social Class (Kuppuswamy Scale)

Socio economic class	*Male frequency*	*%*	*Female Frequency*	*%*	*Total*	*%*
I	3	3.94	—	—	3	3.94
II	3	3.94	3	3.94	6	7.88
III	29	38.17	21	27.64	50	65.81
IV	13	17.11	4	5.26	17	22.37
V	—	—	—	—	—	—
Total	48	63.16	28	36.84	76	100.00

Table II
Distribution of diarrhoeal cases according to literacy status of mothers of patients, number of persons in the family and overcrowding in the houses

Literacy status of Mothers of patients	*Illeterate* 32 (42.10%)	*Primary* 25 (32.89%)	*Middle* 8 (10.53%)	*Secondary* 7 9.21%)	*Higher* 4 (5.27%)	*Total* 76 (10%)
Number of persons in the family	4 of less than 4 55 (72.35%)		5-6 persons (25.00%)	More than 6 persons 2 (2.64%)		76 (100%)
		(z = 3.89 P < 0.05)				
Over crowding in the house	Present 56 (73.68%)		Absent (26.32%)	–	–	76 (100%)
		(z = 4.12 P < 0.05)				

Table III
Distribution of diarrhoeal cases with associated signs and symptoms

Signs and Symptoms	*Number of cases*	*Percentage*
Dehydration	60	78.95
Fever	57	75.00
Vomitting	56	73.68
Pain abdomen	18	23.68
Acidosis	6	7.90
Suppression of urine	3	3.94
CNS Symptoms	3	3.94

Due to multiplicity of signs and symptoms, the total percentage in the above table is more than 100.

Table IV
Distribution of diarrhoeal cases as per feeding pattern dehydration status grades of malnutrition up to the age 24 months

Age Groups in months	*0-5*	*6-11*	*12-23*	*Total*	*Grand Total*
Feeding pattern					
(a) Breast fed	7 (13.20)	4 (7.56)	–	11 (20.75)	
(b) Top fed	–	2 (3.78)	3 (5.66)	5 (9.43)	53 (100)
(c) Mixed fed	–	12 (22.64)	25 (47.17)	37 (69.82)	
Dehydration Status					
(a) No Dehydration	–	3 (5.66)	5 (7.56)	7 (13.20)	
(b) Mild	2 (3.78)	6 (11.32)	12 (22.64)	20 (37.72)	53 (100)
(c) Moderate	2 (3.78)	9 (16.99)	8 (15.00)	19 (35.88)	
(d) Severe	3 (5.66)	2 (3.78)	2 (3.78)	7 (13.20)	
Malnutrition Grades					
'O'	1 (1.88)	4 (7.56)	11 (20.75)	16 (30.70)	
'I'	5 (9.44)	10 (18.87)	11 (20.75)	26 (48.76)	53 (100)
'II'	–	4 (7.56)	3 (51.66)	7 (13.20)	
'III'	1 (1.88)	1 (1.88)	1 (1.88)	3 (5.66)	
'IV'	–	1 (1.88)	–	1 (1.88)	

Percentage in parenthesis

Table V
Distribution of diarrhoeal cases as per isolation of causative agents from stools

Agents	*Frequency*	*Percentage*
Salmonella	3	3.95
Shigeila	3	3.95
Camphylobacter Jejuni	4	5.26
Yersina enterocolitica	1	1.31
Staphylococcus Aureus	2	2.63
Ascaris lumbricoldes	8	10.54
Giardia Lamblia	6	7.89
Entamoeba Hystolytica	1	1.31
No Isolation	48	63.16
	76	100.00

Table VI
Distribution of diarrhoeal cases by knowledge attitude and practice of Oral Rehydration Therapy by mothers of patients

KAP BY MOTHERS OF PATIENTS	
Knowledge about ORT	38 out of 76
Attitude towards ORT	12 out of 38
Practice of ORT	10 out of 12

Discussion

As per present study, majority of cases (63.81%) belonged to social class III followed by social class IV (22.37%). This difference was found to be statistically highly significant ($p < 0.001$). Shakuntala and Urmil, (5) Srivastava et al (6) and Bhai et al (7) also concluded from their studies that there was a definite association between, social class and incidence of diarrhoea. The higher incidence of diarrhoea in lower socio economic groups may be due to varied social factors such as ignorance, lack of health eduction, overcrowding, poor hygiene, malnutrition, illiteracy etc.

The present study revealed that incidence of diarrhoea was inversely proportional to the literacy status of mothers. Similar findings were observed by Shakuntala and Urmil (5) and Saran et al (8). The higher incidence of diarrhoea among children of illitrate mothers could be due to their lack of health eduction reflected in their poor personal hygienc and inadequate hygeinic practices.

As per present study, more cases of diarrhoea were from families consisiting of 4 or less than 4 members. However Amanullah (9) and Srivastava (10) found that the incidence of diarrhoea was more in families having 5 or more members. Idris et al (11) on the other hand could not find any association between the size of the family and incidence of diarrhoea. The exact reason responsible for more number of cases in small families as per present study is not known.

The present study brings out an association between diarrhoeal diseases and overcrowding in the house. Similar observations were also made by Saran et al (8), Srivastava (10), and Srivastava et al (6) in their studies at Varanasi, Lucknow and Kanpur respectively.

The present study revealed that dehydration and fever were present in 78.95 per cent and 75.00 per cent cases respectively. Studies by other workers also revealed that dehydration was predominently present in most cases followed by fever. For example, Srivastava et al (6,12) Ghai and Kumar (13) found dehydration to be present in 79.80%, 99.80% and 68.80% cases and fever in 40.00% 48.20% and 25.30% cases respectively. It cannot be overemphasised that dehydration should be watched and combated in all cases of diarrhoea.

According to findings of present study, out of 53 cases of diarrhoea who were less than 24 months of age, 20.75 per cent were exclusively breast fed, 79.25 per cent were top fed and or received mixed fed. These findings are in conformity with those of Amanullah (9) and Santha Krishnan et al (14) whose studies revealed that diarrhoea affected 20% of exclusively breast fed children. It is generally accepted that breast milk possesses immunological properties and breast fed babies suffer less from infective diarrhoeas than bottle fed babies.

Majority of diarrhoeal cases (67-92%) were found to be suffereing from malnutrition of different grades in the present study. More or less similar findings were observed by Achar (15), Srivastavas et al (12) and Shakuntala and Urmil (5).

In the present study, isolation of pathogenic organisms could be achieved from 36.84% cases only. 19.74% cases had parasitic infestations and 17.10% had bacterial infections. Saran et al (8) also reported a higher prevalence of parasitic infestations (43.27%) where as Miglani et al (16) observed a lower prevalence of parasitic infestations (9.00%) in their studies at Varanasi and Bikaner respectively.

The present study brought out that 50 per cent mothers of the patients, had no knowledge about ORT and out of those who had knowledge only 26.32 per cent were practicing it. In their community based study in Delhi slums, Shakuntala and Urmil (5) found that only 20.20 per cent mothers had knowledge about ORT out of which 47.90 per cent practised it at home to prevent dehydration in their children suffering from diarrhoea.

The study thus brought out necessity of greater emphasis on health education of mothers particularly regarding ORT, it's role in prevention of dehydration and how to prepare and adminster it to children suffering from diarrhoea.

References

1. Mathur R. Aetiology of Gastroenteritis in Children. Proceeding of the Nutrition Society of India 1981; 31:17.
2. Park JE, Park K. Text book of Preventive and Social Medicine, 11thed M/s Banarsidas Bhanot Jabalpur 1986 : 191.
3. Diarrhoeal diseases. Bull ICMR 1984; 14:1
4. Kuppuswamy B. Manual of Socio Economic Status Scale (Urban). Manasyan, 32 Netaji Subhash Marg, Delhi-6.
5. Shakuntala B, Urmil D. Diarrhoeal disease morbidity in children below 5 years in Urban slums of Delhi. Ind J Med Res 1986; 84: 54-58.

6. Srivastava JR, Verma V., Garg BG. Acute Diarrhoea in childhood. Indian Paediatr 1968; 35: 217-44.

7. Ghai OP, Kalra SL, Jaiswal VN. Epidemiology of diarrhoea in infants and preschool children in a rural community areas Delhi; Indian paediatr 1969; 6:.

8. Saran M. Gaur SD. Verma BL, Arun Kumar. An Epidemiological study of Diarrhoea among children under 5 years of age in a slum community. Indian Paediatr 1979; 16: 33-39.

9. Amanullah, quoted by Srivastava et al. A clinical and Actiological study of Diarrhoea in Hospitalised Children at Lucknow, Ind J Med Res 1973; 61; 596-602.

10. Srivastava AK. A Socio Medical study of children upto 3 yrs of age suffering from Diarrhoea. Admitted in children hospital KG Medical College Lucknow. A thesis submitted for MD (PSM) Lucknow University.

11. Indris MZ, Saxena SC, Malik GK, Srivastava BC. Feeding practices and diarrhoeal Episodes among Rural and Urban infants of Lucknow. Indian Paediatr 1981: 18 : 311-16.

12. Srivastava AK; Bhatnagar JK. Prasad BG, Sharma NL. A clinical and Actiological study of Diarrhoea in Hospitalised children at Lucknow. Ind J Med Res 1973; 61: 596-602.

13. Ghai OP, Kumar V, Diarrhoea in infants and children. Ind J paediatr 1969 : 262.

14. Shantana Krishnan BR; Thangadoral C Moses LG, Balgopal RV. Bacteriological study of Acute Gastro-enterities in hospitalised children Ind Paediatr 1974; 11 : 653-55.

15. Achar ST. Paediatrics in developing Tropical countries. Orient Longman Ltd. 1978; 381 : 156.

16. Miglani N, Lohra UK; Gupta BD. Bacteriological, Mycological and Parasitological study in childhood diarrhoea in Bikaner Ind Paediatr 1979; 16 : 569-75.

Chapter-3

Medico-Social Profile of Male Teenager STD Patients

Abstract

A medico-social study of 250 STD patients attending a clinic was undertaken in late 80s. A brief analysis was done in respect of age, literacy status, source and type of infection among the study subjects. The findings, have pointed to the importance of imparting health education to the teenagers, specially more among illiterate persons.

Introduction

Sexually transmitted diseases (STD) are the only group of communicable diseases which have defied the control measures even in the most developed countries. The World Health Organisation (WHO) has accorded priority to STD next only to malaria and tuberculosis (Nair et al, 1973). The rising incidence of STD particularly among the teenagers has become the cause of serious concern all over the world. These diseases are multifcatorial in their etiology and their prevalence in any community depends on various socio-economic factors. Biological and psychological changes associated with marked desire for sexual adventures during adolescene have put the teenagers in a 'high risk' group. During modern times, rapid urbanisation and industrialisation had not only broken down the established class structure but also shattered the social and religious constraints which prevented promiscuous sexual behaviour. A WHO report in 1977 noted with concern the striking increase in the incidence of STD among teengar group. In India a few surveys carried out earlier indicated that STD among teenagers had already posed serious medico-social problem (Singh 1962, Saha 1979, Singh 1979, Bhattacharjee 1979, Dongre 1975). In view of the foregoing, this study was undertaken to determine the medico-social profile of male teenagar patients attending a STD clinic in Pune.

Material and Method

The present study was carried out during April-August 1987 at STD clinic of Dr Kotnis Arogya Kendra under Municipal Corporation of Pune. This clinic is located close to main red light area of the city. During the period of study, a total of 1624 patients attended the clinic, out of them 285 were teenagers (17.55%). Among them 250 were male subjects. Relevant information was collected in a pretested schedule through interview technique.

Result and Discussion

Age distributiion of cases. This is show in table.

Table 1
Distribution of male teenager STD cases according to age

Age in years	*Cases*	*Percentage*
13	1	0.40
14	1	0.40
15	11	4.40
16	22	8.80
17	28	11.20
18	95	38.00
19	92	36.80
Total	250	100.00

It is evident from table 1 that maximum number of teenagers were 18 to 19 years old (74.80%). This could be because of increasing sexual activity during the adolescence, financial freedom, increasing friends circle and greater yearning among teenagers to become independent and explore the world in their own way.

Diagnosis of the cases

It is obvious from table 2 that gonorrhoea was the most frequently diagnosed STD (37.60%), followed by chancroid (36.00%). Dongre and Advent (1975) in their study of STD patients among students in Pune, found a very high percentage of chancroid (76.00%) followed by gonorrhoea (15.50%), syphilis (3.50%), combination of syphilis and soft sore (3.0%) and LGV (3.0%).

Table 2
Distribution of teenager STD cases according to diagnosis

Diagnosis	*Cases*	*Percentage*
Syphilis primary	28	11.40
Syphilis secondary	2	0.80
Gonorrhoea	94	37.60
Chancroid	90	36.00
LGV	8	3.20
Balano-prosthitis	12	4.80
Herpes genitalis	7	2.80
Condyloma acuminata	9	3.60
Total	250	100.00

Marital Status: Only 2 male teenagers (0.80%) were married and rest 99.20 percent were bachelors in the study population.

Distribution according to religion

Hindu teenagers accounted for 84.00 percent cases. Next in order were Budhists (8.00%), Muslims (7.20%) and Christians (0.80%).

Family background

Table 3 shows that the almost half of the cases were from nuclear families (49.20%). The cases, when classified according to urban/rural background and the type of family, revealed that the proportion of nuclear and three generation families with urban background was more as compared to the rural background and this difference was found to be statistically significant ($p < 0.001$).

Table 3
Distribution of cases according to type of family and urban/rural background

	Type of family				
Back-ground	*Joint*	*Nuclear*	*Three Generation*	*Staying alone*	*Total*
Urban	37 (19.47%)	98 (51.58%)	7 (3.68%)	190 (100.00%)	
Rural	13 (21.67%)	25 (41.67%)	8 (13.33%)	14 (23.33%)	60 (100.00%)
Total	50 (20.00%)	123 (49.20%)	56 (22.40%)	21 (8.40%)	250 (100.00%)

X : 24,84; df : 3; $p < 0.001$

Literary Status : This is depicted in Table 4.

It is seen from table 4 that 82 percent teenagers were literate and 18 percent illiterate. Bhattacharjee et al (1979) in Delhi found that illiterates contributed the highest number of cases (60.20%), while Gokhale et al (1972) in Pune observed that most of the cases were unable to read or write. The findings of the present study are similar to those of Seth (1979) who reported 17 per cent illiterate and 62 percent educated upto school level. 31.20 percent of teenagers in the present study were still pursuing their studies.

Table 4

Distribution of cases according to education status

Education	*Cases*	*Percentage*
Intermediate and above	12	4.80
High school and above	44	17.60
6th to 9th standard	104	41.60
Above 9th standard	45	18.00
Illiterate	45	18.00
Total	250	100.00

Occupation

Table 5 reveals that financially independent teengers (comprising of skilled, semi-skilled and unskilled workers) contributed 57.20 percent of the total cases. Financially dependents on the other hand (students and unemployed) contributed 42.00 percent of the total cases. The present study compares favourably with the findings of Nair et al (1979), Saha et al (1979) and Sidhu et al (1979) who found a higher percentage of unskilled workers.

This shown in Table 5.

Table 5

Distribution of the cases according to occupation

Occupation	*Cases*	*Percentage*
Student	78	31.20
Skilled worker	3	1.20
Semi skilled worker	33	13.20
Unskilled worker	107	42.00
Unemployed	29	11.60
Total	250	100.00

Knowledge and experience about first sexual intercourse

The persent study revealed that by 14 years of age, 85.20 percent knew about the sexual intercourse and 64.80 percent had their first sexual experience between 15 to 18 years of age. Curiosity was mentioned as the main reason for first sexual intercourse by 46 percent of teenagers, followed by persuation by friends (34.03%) and excessive sex desire (10.40%). Other reasons mentioned were - influence of films, pornographic literature, persuation/allurement by sexual partners.

Table 6

Distribution of cases according to source of present infection and number of

Number of sexual experience	*Experience of Sexual Act* *Source of present infection* *Prostitutes*	*Amateur*	*Total*
First time	61 (69.32%)	27 (30.68%)	88 (100.00%)
More than once	145 (89.50%)	17 (10.50%)	162 (100.00%)
Total	206 (82.40%)	44 (17.60%)	250 (100.00%)

X^2 : 16.02; df : 1; $p < 0.001$

It is evident that patients with more than one exposure were having less of psychological inhibition and therefore got exposed to readily available prostitutes. On further classifying cases according to number of sexual experience, it is observed that among repeaters, prostitutes were source of infection in 89.50 percent cases while among first time exposures, they were source of infection in only 69.32 percent cases and this difference is found statistically significant ($p < 0.001$).

Knowledge of STD.

This is shown in Table 7.

Table 7 reveals that only 13.60 percent of teenagers had correct knowledge about mode of acquiring STD. 22 percent had wrong knowledge and 64.40 percent had no knowledge at all. However, education standard and status of knowledge about mode of acquiring STD when statistically analysed showed that the difference was not significant ($p > 0.05$).

Table 7
Distribution of cases according to educational standard and status of knowledge about mode of acquiring STD

Educational standard	*Knowledge about mode of acquiring STD*			
	Correct knowledge	*Wrong knowledge*	*No knowledge*	*Total*
Intermediate and above	3 (25.00%)	2 (16.76%)	7 (58.33%)	12 (100.00%)
High school and above	8 (18.18%)	10 (22.73%)	26 (59.09%)	44 (100.00%)
6 - 9th standard	12 (11.54%)	17 (16.35%)	75 (72.11%)	104 (100.00%)
Up to 5th standard	4 (8.89%)	13 (28.98%)	28 (62.22%)	45 (100.00%)
Illiterate	7 (15.55%)	13 (28.89%)	25 (55.56%)	45 (100.00%)
Total	34 (13.60%)	55 (22.00%)	161 (64.40%)	250 (100.00%)

X : 5.06; df : 4; $p > 0.05$

Note: Rows 1,2 and 3,4 have been clubbed for statistical analysis.

Knowledge about prophylaxis

This study also revealed that only 5.60 percent had correct knowledge about prophylactics. 80.80 percent had no knowledge and 13.60 percent had wrong knowledge. Various misconceptions among teenagers about prophylaxis were scrubbing the penis with dry cloth or application of urine after intercourse, avoiding sexual act with menstruating woman and having intercourse only with good looking prostitutes as they were supposed to be free from infection.

Other interesting findings

More than three-fourth of the study subjects committed sexual intercourse in brothels. Other places, mentioned were ether partner's house, friends' house, open places, hotel/lodge, abandoned houses and even public lavatory in one case. Except two prostitutes who lured the teenagers for sexual act, all others were paid in cash ranging for Rs. 1.00 to Rs. 21.00. Of amateurs, majority did not receive any payment; however some of them were paid in terms of kind (meal or gifts). Majority of the cases (80.80%) had a feeling of guilt after acquiring the disease whereas this proportion was found to be still higher (90.59%) among those acquired infection following first sexual exposure.

Summary

A study of 250 male teenager STD cases was carried out to determine the association between certain medico-social factors e.g. age, type of infection, educational status, source of infection, knowledge about mode of acquiring infection and prophylaxis etc. Salient findings of the study such as gonorrhoea being the commonest type of STD, curiosity being the main reason for first sexual exposure and prostitutes being the major source of infection have been highlighted in this communication.

Acknowledgment

The authors are grateful to the Commissioner and Health Officer of Pune Municipal Corporation for according permission to carry out the study at Dr. Kotnis Arogya Kendra, Gadikhana, Pune and to the staff of the clinic for extending the facilities and necessary co-operation.

Reference

1. Nair BKH, Viswan MP, Venugopal DS, Nair PS. (1973) An epidemiological study of venereal diseases. Indian J Med Res, 6: 1967.

2. World Health Organisation. (1977) Health needs of adolescents. WHO Tech Rep Ser No. 609.

3. Swasth Hind (1971; '5 : 207).

4. Singh R. (1962) Pattern of venereal diseases, Indian J Venereal Dermatol 1962; 28 : 62.

5. Saha PC, Ghosh BN, Datta AK. (1979) A study on sociodemographic characteristies and knowledge about VD of male STD patients attending a treatment centre in Calcutta and their contact. Indian J Pub Hlth 23 : 44-56. 1962; 28 : 62.

6. Singh JV, Narayan V. (1979) Concomittant venereal infections in male patients attending a VD clinic at Lucknow. Indina J. Med Res 70 : 928.

7. Bhattacharjee SK, Singh R, Sharma RC. (1979) Ecology of early syphilis patient : A study of eighty cases. Indian J Dermatol Venereal, 45 : 436

8. Dongre PM, Advent PV (1975) Venereal disease among students. Maharashtra Medical Journal 22 : 47

9. Subhash Babu D, Marwah SM, Singh G. (1976) Social and behaviolural aspects of venereal disease among resident male university students. International J Epid 5 : 121

10. Gokhale BB, Master RS. Gokhale T.B. (1972) The clients of the common prostitutes. Indian J Dermatol Venereal, 38 : 243.

11. Seth T.R. Socio-physical factors and incidence of VD. (1970) Indian J Dermatol Venereal 36 : 93.

12. Prasad BG. (1970) Social classificasion. J Indian MA 55 : 193.

13. Hiramani AB, Srivastava U, Misra RS. (1981) STD patients in a New Delhi Hospital; An action research study. Swasth Hind 25 : 186.

14. Sidhu CMS, Mahajan RC, Srivastava BC. (1969) A socio-medical study of VD cases in two industrial cities. Antiseptic, 66 : 843.

Chapter–4

Customs and Beliefs About Small Pox

Abstract

This study was undertaken in few villages in Gwalior district in midsixties much before eradication of the dreaded disease "Smallpox". In the medico-social study, only an attempt was made to analyse the respondents' views about causation, mode of spread and preventive measures against small pox. The study highlighted the scope and importance of health education, specially to allay the mis-belief against vaccination and then ultimately achieving the success in eradicating the disease from surface of the earth once for all.

Introduction

Following independence, India had launched eradication programmes against the two communicable diseases - malaria and smallpox. Smallpox theoretically was easier to eradicate by systematic vaccination and re-vaccination of the human herd. This was an accomplished fact in many developed countries. But the same could not be said about the smallpox eradication programme in India. Although significant improvements had taken place in the conquest of smallpox, but ultimately conquest was achieved only in 1977. The reason for the succcess or failure of a health programme is to be found in the public cooperation, which in turn depends upon the public attitude, customs and beliefs.

During the course of an assessment in mid sixties, of the National Smallpox Eradication Programme in Gwalior district, Madhya Pradesh, the author collected data pertaining to the customs and beliefs of the people about smallpox in that part of the country. Four villages namely, Hastinapur, Mohanpur, Jaduria and Maharajpur were taken up near Gwalior city but situated in different directions varying from 2 to 20 miles from Gwalior. From each village, about 125 people above the age of 15 years covering all age, sex and social groups were interviewed at random by a carefully prepared schedule. In all,500 people were interviewed. Their opinion, beliefs and customs are summarised in the tables that follows and are discussed seriatim.

Findings

1. Cause of Smallpox

It is well known that rural people in India had divergent views about the causation of smallpox. The views of the people in Gwalior region are given below in Table1.

Table 1
Views of the people about the causation of smallpox

Causes		*No. of persons responding*	*Percent*
1.	Godess (Mata)	296	39.2
2.	Uncleanliness	222	44.4
3.	Bad air	189	37.8
4.	Germs	158	31.6
5.	Not aware	95	19.0
6.	Bad health	49	9.8
7.	Karma	46	9.2
8.	Fatalistic	38	7.6

Many respondents gave more than one answer

It will be seen from Table 1, that the majority of the people (59 percent) held the views that smallpox was caused by Mata * (Deitistie Theory of disease). Survey carried out by Bharara (1961, 1962) in Uttar Pradesh had also shown that 55.8 percent of people believed in the 'deitistic theory'. The fact that people held more than one view about the causation of smallpox indicated that they were not clear in their minds about the cause of smallpox. Here is an area for health education of the people. Dissemination of correct information about the causation of smallpox was thought to be most important step in the eradication of the disease.

2. Age and Sex Occurrence

80 percent of the study subjects felt that small pox was more a disease of children than of adults. In this, they were correct as it was one of common observation and experience. Some were of the opinion (86%) that the disease was more frequent in females than in males.

3. Seasonal Incidence

The majority of people (68.4%) mentioned that the disease occurred mostly during summer season. Some said (25.2%) that the disease occurred in any season. In this, the people were not far from the truth, Epidemics of smallpox occurred mostly in the summer months, whereas cases kept occuring throughout the year.

4. Differentiation from Chickenpox

81.8 percent of the people mentioned that if rashes were bigger in size and abundant all over the body, it was one of smallpox. 13.2 percent of the people were of the opinion that smallpox was a more serious disease than chickenpox. Suffice it to say, that people confused chickenpox for smallpox. An attack of chickenpox after vaccination often shook their faith in vaccination. Health education on this aspect also would be beneficial and would help to overcome some of the misconceptions and prejudices, people had about smallpox.

5. Complications of Smallpox

People were aware, to some extent, of the complications. It is true that smallpox was one of the leading causes of blindness in India. 33.4 percent said that the disease disfigured and 56.4 percent of the people said that the disease was fatal. This indicated that people were aware of the ill effects of smallpox.

6. Prevention of Smallpox

Study subjects were asked if they knew how smallpox could be prevented. It was encouraging to find that 66.4 percent of the interviewes another said that smallpox could be prevented by vaccination. In a survey carried out in 1964, by K.P. Srivastava and K.N. Maurya in Uttar Pradesh, only 15 percent of the population believed in efficiencyof vaccination. This was an interesting finding in that although the majority of people (59.2%) believed that the disease was due to the influence of Mata, they also believed (66.4%) that vaccination prevented smallpox. This is because, people acquired faith in vaccination as had been in vogue in India,for the last 100 years or so. A good majority of the people were convinced about the usefulness of vaccination.

7. Age of Vaccination

The majority of people, i.e. (79%) were of the opinion that primary vaccination should be done within the first year of life, 39 per cent favoured vaccination between 6 to 12 months. Thus the climate of opinion was favourable for the vaccination of infants and children.

8. Revaccination

People were ingnorant about the need for periodic revaccination. 43.2 percent of the people considered that vaccination performed once was enough for life long protection where as 56.8 percent expressed that revaccination at certain intervals might be necessary. Thus there were divergent views among the people about the need for revaccination. Since eradication of smallpox was the ultimate goal, the need for effective health education of people on this aspect, had to be over-emphasised. Here was another important area for health education of the people.

9. Antivaccinationists

5 percent of the people interviewed were against vaccination. An attempt was made to find out the reasons why they were against vaccination. The reasons given by them are shown table below:-

Table II

Reasons Against Vaccination

Reasons	*Number*	*Percent*
Fear of physical or mental harm	11	2.2
Incapacitation	4	0.8
Previous bad experience	4	0.8
Cannot explain	3	0.6
Mistrust and lack of faith	2	0.4
Leads to sterility	1	0.2
Total	25	5

It is worthwhile to note that none of the reasons given by the anti-vaccinationists had any bearing upon religious beliefs. Thus, the situatioin was favourable for persuading the anti-vaccinationists to accept vaccination, without infringing upon their religious beliefs.

10. Some customs and practices

It was found that people adopted a number of measures when there was a case of smallpox in a family. About 56.6

percent of people said that it was necessary to worship the Goddess 'Sheetla Mata'. Shaving and cutting hair was not to be undertaken by the members of the affected family according to 66 percent of the study subjects. About 40 percent of the people said that frying of food in fats and oils and use of aromatic condiments should be eschewed. Most of the people, (82%) expressed great faith in Neem leaves. Some advocated bath with Neem leaves; others said that Neem leaves should be burnt in the affected house. Some people said that there should be a small fire made out of cowdung cakes, kept constantly burning in the room of the patient; the idea was to keep away the evil spirits from the house. If there was a case of smallpox, 67.4 percent of people said that they would not visit the affected family. 84.2 percent of people said that the patients should be isolated, and none should be allowed to cast his or her shadow on the patient excepting those who attended or nursed the case.

A common practice in the rural areas was not to notify when there was smallpox, lest they should incur the wrath of the Goddess. In the survey, 56.4 percent of the people said that they would not tell others, if there was a case of smallpox in the family, thus resulting in disastrous out breaks of smallpox epidemics. About 6.4 percent of the people said that vaccination should not be accepted by the members of the affected family, till the worship of Mata was over. If contacts are not vaccinated early, there would be more cases of smallpox.

Regarding the disposal of the dead, it was interesting to observe that although 87.8 percent of the people were Hindus whose custom was to cremate the dead, they said they would have the dead body of smallpox buried rather than burnt. They expressed that in the process of burning the smallpox germs might vitiate the atmosphere. About 0.6 percent of the people said that the bodies of smallpox should be thrown in the river.

Conclusion

The study threw light on the several factors with special regard to beliefs, customs and practices which was involved in epidemiology of smallpox. An understanding of these factors was essential for eradication of smallpox. People had conflicting views about the cause, mode of spread and prevention of disease. Much of this, no doubt was due to ignorance and illiteracy of the people. Though most of the people believed in vaccination, but they also believed in 'Deitistic' theory. Since the customs and beliefs guided their action and practices, health education of the people assumed great importance in successful implementation of National Smallpox Eradication Programme (NSEP)

An intensive health education drive always preceded the mass vaccination drive.

In course of an educational programme, beliefs which were scientifically beneficial e.g. isolation, disinfection, usefulness of vaccination, were to be encouraged, but other beliefs and practices which had harmful effects should be discouraged. The health education drive, which should be made a 'people's programme were to be done by increasing involvement of Pradhans, panchayat members and other influential persons of the community. Public health workers with help of workers from Education and related departments should integrate the principles and technique of health education and avail every oportunity to persuade and convince the people about the utility of the vaccination. The survey had also pointed out that the individual approach in earning cooperation of the people for participation in public health programme, e.g. mass vaccinatioin drive, was most effective; the next being the group approach. So public health workers in their respective areas were to disseminate health education and contact leaders first to prepare the ground for the success of the programme. Every effort was to be made to ensure that educational and publicity programmes go simultaneously.

References

1. Bharara S.S. (1961) Public attitude in relation to smallpox; Health Education Bureau, Lucknow (UP)

2. Idem (1962) People's beliefs and attitudes on smallpox; Swasth Hind Vol-VI

3. Dutta P.K. (1965) The evaluation of NSEP in Gwalior distt. Unpublished thesis submitted of MD (Prev. Med) of Jiwaji University P-128.

4. K.P. Srivastava (1964) Report of study into Acceptance of smallpox Vaccination & K.N. Maurya, Health Education Bureau, UP, Lucknow.

SECTION II

NON-COMMUNICABLE DISEASES

Chapter–5

Medico-Social Profile of the Institutional Blind

Abstract

A medico-social study of 196 institutionalised blind individuals was undertaken for a period of six months in Pune. Distribution of study population according to some of the underlying causes and their relationship to the various social determinants have been discussed in this paper. Two third of the study subjects suffered from the present disability either due to infection, malnutrition or accidents which were preventable to a great extent.

Introduction

According to a WHO estimate, there are 28 million blind people in the world. In India, there are about 9 million blind people and about 45 million visually handicapped. The prevalence of blindness in India is estimated to be 1.5 percent of the population. (1) Thirty percent of the blind in India lose their eye sight before they attain 21 years of age and that too, most cases during the first 5 years of life. (2) In a developing country like India, the problem of blindness is further compounded by social factors like poverty, illiteracy and lack of education and medical facilities. To appreciate the phenomenon of blindness more comprehensively, one must understand not only the medical aspects of this malady but also the impact of it's socio-economic determinants. Keeping this view in mind, the study of medico-social profile of institutionalised blind was undertaken. Some of the salient findings of this study are highlighted in this article.

Material and Methods

This study was carried out in two institutions for the blind in Pune, namely (i) Technical Training Institute of Poona, which imparts vocational training to 100 blind men and women aged 18-40 years but without any residential facility, and (ii) Poona School and Home for the Blind Boys which imparts formal education to 100 blind boys aged 6-18 years and provide residential facilities.

The study was carried out for a priod of six month in 1986. A pretested schedule was used to record the findings of the interview and examination of the subjects. The schedule was devised in consultation with the Ophthalmologist of Armed Forces Medical College , Pune. In case of difficulty, the cases were referred to the Ophthalmologist at Command hospital, Pune for expert examination and diagnosis. Socio-economic status of head of the family was assessed according to the scale devised. (3) In case of children, if any information was not forthcoming, the same was obtained from the school authorities.

Findings and Discussion

Study Population: A total number of 196 blind subjects formed the study population. Their age were ranging from 6 to 40 years. 93 percent of the study population was male, giving a male and female ratio of 13:1. They belonged to two religions only i.e. Hindu (190 subjects) and Muslims (6 subjects). Educationwise 25 subjects were totally illiterate; 91 educated upto primary school level; 33 upto middle school level; 43 upto high school level; 3 upto higher secondary level and only 1 upto graduate level. Thus, 87 percent of the study subjects were literate.

Study Population and Social Class: Distribution of study population according to social class is shown in Table1. The Table reveals that two third of the subjects were from lower social class and there was a gradual increase in proportion of the study population with lowering of social status. It is a well established fact that people from lower socio-economic status have higher prevalence of blindness. The findings of other epidemiological studies of the institutionalised blind also observed that higher proportion of subjects belonged to lower socio-economic status. (4, 5, 6).

Table 1
Distribution of Study Population According to Social Class

Social Class	*Number*	*Percentage*
I	3	1.53
II	20	10.20
III	43	21.94
IV	129	65.82
V	1	0.51
Total	196	100.00

Urban-Rural-Distribution: This is depicted in Table 2. Majority of the study population was urban with an urban and rural ratio of 1.76 : 1. A study conducted in Orissa in 1976 showed higher prevalence of blindness in urban area (Urban 3.6 percent and rural 2.2 percent. (7) However, National Sample Survey in 1981 revealed a higher prevalence of blindness in rural areas both at national level and at the Maharashtra State Level. (8) But the findings of the present study compares favourably with the findings of the study of the institutionalised blind. (6)

Table 2
Urban/Rural Distribution of the Study Population

	Number	*Percentage*
Urban	125	63.78
Rural	71	36.22
Total	196	100.00

Causes of Blindness: Distribution of study population according to causes of blindness is shown in Table 3. It is evident from this table that infections constituted the most important group of causes of blindness (44.39%) and alongwith nutritional causes, accidents, injuries and toxemias of pregnancies accounted for almost two third of the blindness in the study population which was preventable. Congenital and hereditary causes accounted for almost one third (32.65%) cases of blindness. In 4.56 percent of cases, the cause could not be ascertained and they were put in the group of 'not known' aetiology. The findings of the present study compare favourably with those of the study of the institutionalised blind. (6) The findings of the other studies could not be compared with the present one due to different modality of classification of the causes of blindness.

Table 3
Causes of Blindness in the Study Population

Sr. No.	*Causes of Blindness*	*Number*	*Percentage*
1.	Congenital	47	23.98
2.	Hereditary	17	8.67
3.	Infections	87	44.39.
4.	Nutritional	29	14.80
5.	Accidents/injuries	6	3.06
6.	Others (Toxaemia of pregnancy)	1	0.51
7.	Not Known	9	4.59
	Total	196	100.00

Ocular Lesions according to Anatomial Location:

Distribution of the study population with reference to this factor is given in Table 4. It is clear that the anterior segment of the eye which is easily accessible to examination and hence whose lesions are potentially preventable by early detection and treatment, was the seat of lesion in approximately 56 percent of cases. The findings of the other studies however show a wide variation in the distribution of anatomical locations of ocular lesions. (6,9)

Table 4
Ocular Lesions According to Anatomical Location

S.No.	Ocular Lesions	No. of Cases	Percentage
1.	Corneal pathology	89	45.41
2.	Lenticular lesions	21	10.72
3.	Retinopathies	22	11.22
4.	Lesions of the optic nerve	6	3.06
5.	Intracranial optic pathways and brain	4	2.04
6.	Bulbar atrophy (phthisis)	35	17.86
7.	Microphthalmos/Anophthalmos	19	9.69
	Total	196	100.00

Distribution of the Blind according to Category of Visual Impairment: From Table 5 it is obvious that more than a third of the subjects had no perception of light at all. Almost 95 percent of the study population qualified for the definition of 'blindness' with 3//60 or less visual acuity and 100 percent of them for 'legal blindness' (visual acuity 6/60 or less). It was, however, observed in other study that 93 percent of the blind belonging to category 5 of visual disability as against only about 36 percent in the present study and 4 percent belonging to category 4 as against 39 percent in the present study. (6)

Table 5
Distribution of the Blind According to Category of Visual Impairment

SNo.	Category of Visual Disability	Number	Percentage
1.	1 (6/18 to 6/60)	—	—
2.	2 (6/60 to 3/60)	11	5.61
3.	3 (3/60 to 1/60)	39	19.90
4.	4 (1/60 to light perception)	76	38.78
5.	5 (No light perception)	70	35.71
6.	(Undetermined/unspecified)	—	—
	Total	196	100.00

Causes in Relation to Age of Onset: It is evident from Table 6 that one third of the subject were blind at the time of birth and among the remaining, most the them acquired blindness before school going age. The findings of the present study compare favourably with other studies. (5,9) However, in another study it was observed that 25 percent of the subjects had onset of blindness before 15 years of age and 55 percent beyond 39 years. (5) Since, maximum age of the subjects in the present study was less than 40 years, the findings cannot be compared with those observed in general population (including elderly above 40 years of age). (5)

Table 6
Causes of Blindness in Relation to Age of Onset
(In years)

Causes	*At Birth*	*1-5*	*6-10*	*11-15*	*16-25*	*26 and above*	*Total*
Congenital	47	-	-	-	-	-	47 (23.98)
Hereditary	17	-	-	-	-	-	17 (8.67)
Infections	-	69	14	4	-	-	87 (44. 39)
Nutritional	-	25	4	-	-	-	29 (14.80)
Accidents/injuries	-	1	2	2	1	-	6 (3.06)
Others (Toxaemia of pregnancy)	-	-	-	-	-	1	1 (0.51)
Not known	-	5	2	1	1	-	9 (4.59)
Total	64	100	22	7	2	1	196 (100)

Causes of Blindness in Relation to Sex: It is clear from Table 7 that congenital causes accounted for higher proportion of blindness among male subjects compared to their female counterparts whereas hereditary causes were found only among the male subjects in the present study. Infections and nutritional causes were seen more among female subjects and the findings are consistent with the findings of other studies. Application of Kajal/Surma and smoke in the kitchen may be attributed to higher proportion of blindness due to infections among female subjects. Similarly malnutrition is more prevalent among females in India and may be responsible for occurrence of higher proportion of nutritional blindness among them. Accidents and injuries accounted for about 3 percent blindness among male subjects against nil in female counterparts and may be due to the fact that males are more prone to accidents.

Table 7
Causes of Blindness in Relation to the Sex of the Blind

Sr.No.	*Causes*	*Male*	*Female*	*Total*
1.	Congenital	46 (25.27)	1 (7.41)	47 (23.98)
2.	Hereditary	17 (9.34)	-	17 (8.67)
3.	Infections	79 (43.41)	8 (57.15)	87 (44.39)
4.	Nutritional	25 (13. 74)	4 (28.57)	29 (14.80)
5.	Accidents/injuries	6 (3.30)	-	6 (3.06)
6.	Toxaemia of Pregnancy	-	1 (7.14)	1 (0.51)
7.	Not known	9 (4.94)	-	9 (4.59)
	Total	182 (100)	14 (100)	196 (100)

(Note: Figures in parentheses indicate percentages)

Application of Kajal/Surma and causes of Blindness: This is depicted in Table 8. It is seen that trachoma and conjunctivitis as causes of blindness were significantly associated with the practice of application of Kajal/Surma in the study population. This findings are in confirmity with the knowledge that the certain customs may predispose to ocular infections like conjunctivitis and trachoma. (1)

Table 8
Application of Kajal/Surma and Causes of Blindness

Causes of Blindness	*Application of Kajal / Surma*		
	Yes	*No*	*Total*
Trachoma	5	2	7
Conjunctivitis	5	14	19
Total	10	16	26

p = <0.046 (by exact test for 2 x 2 tables). Significant

Causes of Blindness and Social Status: It is seen that congenital and hereditary causes accounted for higher proportion of blindness among upper and middle social class subjects whereas infections and accident/injuries were responsible for higher proportion of disability among lower social class of study population as shown in Table 9. Statistical analysis showed high significance of the differences in various causes in relation to social status of the subjects. Authors of other studies have also found similar findings to those of the present study. (5) A higher proportion of blindness among people of lower socio-economic status were due to infections.

Table 9
Causes of Blindness In Relation to Social Status

Sr. No.	*Causes*	*Upper & Middle Social Class*	*Lower Social Class*	*Total*
1.	Congenital	21 (31.82)	26 (20.00)	47 (23.98)
2.	Hereditary	12 (18.18)	5 (3.85)	17 (8. 67)
3.	Infections	19 (28.79)	68 (52.31)	87 (44.39)
4.	Nutritional	10 (15.15)	19 (14.61)	29 (14.80)
5.	Accidents/injuries	1 (1.51)	5 (3.85)	6 (3.06)
6.	Toxaemia of Pregnancy	-	1 (0.77)	1 (0.51)
7.	Not known	3 (4.55)	6 (4.61)	9 (4.59)
	Total	66 (100.00)	130 (100.00)	196 (100)

$X^2 = 20.30$ $df < 4$; $p < 0.001$ (Highly significant)

Note: (i) For statistical analysis values at Sr. No. 5, 6 and 7 have been clubbed together.

(ii) Figures in parentheses indicate percentages

Urban/Rural Distribution of Study population and Causes of Blindness: It is seen from Table 10 that different causes were responsible for almost similar proportion of blindness among subjects both from urban and rural areas except in case of accidents/injuries and toxaemia of pregnancy which were not seen in case of rural subjects. There was no statistically significant association between causes of blindness and urban/rural distribution of the study population.

Table 10
Urban/Rural Distribution of Study Population and Causes of Blindness

Sr.No.	Causes	Urban	Rural	Total
1.	Congenital	29 (23.20)	18 (25.35)	47 (23.98)
2.	Hereditary	9 (7.20)	8 (11.27)	17 (8.67)
3.	Infections	57 (45.60)	30(42.26)	87 (44.39)
4.	Hutritional	18 (14.40)	11 (15.49)	29 (14.80)
5.	Accidents/injuries	6 (4.80)	-	6 (3.06)
6.	Toxaemia of Pregnancy	1 (0.80)	-	1 (0.51)
7.	Not known	5 (4.00)	4 (5.63)	9 (4.59)
	Total	125 (100.00)	71 (100.00)	196 (100)

X = 1.89: df > 4 p > 0.5 (not significant)

Note: (i) For statistical analysis values at Sr. No. 5, 6 and 7 have been clubbed together.
(ii) Figures in parentheses indicate percentages

Conclusion

The present study of 196 institutionalised blind subjects has revealed that almost two third blindness was attributable to causes preventable in nature. Proper health education and preventive precautions observed by the individual/parents should have prevented it. A critical analysis of association between certain social factors and causes of blindness revealed a higher proportion of subjects from the lower socio-economic status in whom infections were found to be the most predominant cause. Trachoma and conjunctivitis as causes of blindness were found to be significantly associated with practice of application of Kajal/Surma in the study population. Majority of the subjects were found to have become blind before school going age. Infections and nutritional causes were seen more among female subjects as compared to their male counterparts. No significant association could be ascertained between causes of blindness and urban/rural background or literacy status of the study population.

References

1. Park J.E. and Park K. (1985) Textbook of Preventive and Social Medicine. 10th edn. Jabalpur, M/s. Banarsidas Bhanot.
2. Government of India, Central Health Education Bureu (1986) Swasth Hind. 12: p. 245.
3. Kappuswamy, B. Manual of Socio-economic Status Scale. Manasayan, 32, Netaji Subhash Marg, Delhi-6.
4. Suri, N.K. Mishra, V.N. Mathur, I.S. Singh, J.V. Bhatnagar, N. Singh, R.B. (1984) Prevalence and pattern of blindness in a rural community. Indian Journal of Prevents and Social Medicine, 15:38-41.
5. Sharma, K.L. Prasad, B.G. (1962) An epidemiological study of blindess in Banki Block of Barabanki District (U.P) Indian Journal of Medical Research, 58: p.842-66.
6. Mehta, Shashi (1977) A study of the institutionalised blind in Maharashtra. A dissertation submitted for M.S. (Ophthalmology), University of Poona (unpublished).
7. World Health Organisation (1979) Data on blindness throughout the world. Who Chronicle, 33: p. 275-93.
8. Government of India, National Sample Survey Organisation, Department of Statistics (1983) Report on survey of disabled persons 305: p. 13-22, New Delhi.
9. Madan Mohan (1982) Adrenwala Oration. Indian J. Ophthalmology, 1983, 31:p. 463.

Chapter–6

A Study of Psychosocial Profile of Institutionalised Blind Individuals in Pune

Introduction

To be blind is a real tragedy, for without sight, the world around us is a closed book. Generally speaking, the term 'blind' means a person who has totally lost his eye sight or whose vision is of no practical value for the purpose of reading or in the general activities of living (Mehta, 1983).

According to WHO estimate, there are 28 million blind people in the world. In India, there are about 9 million blind people and about 45 million visually handicapped. 30 percent of them lose their eye sight before they attain 21 years (Park and Park, 1985).

In a developing country like India, this problem is further compounded by social factors like poverty, illiteracy and lack of proper medical facilities. The fact that two thirds of the blind suffer from preventable causes, makes the tragedy even more poignant (Khurana et al. 1973).

Control of blindness has now been included in the Prime Minister's 20 Point Programme and is expected to receive maximum attention. Effective implementation of this programme would help to relieve miseries of a large number of people who live a life not only enveloped in darkness but also in pity and patronage. The prevalence of blindness is expected to be brought down from estimated 1.5 percent to 0.2 percent by turn of the century (Roy, 1984).

The present survey was undertaken to study some of the psychosocial aspects of blind inmates in two institutions. This being a study of the institutionalised blind individuals, it may not reveal the exact magnitude of the problem in general population; yet it should help us to understand complex psychosocial aspects of the blindness and serve as a guide to ameliorate the miseries of affected individuals in future.

Material and Methods

The present study was carried out in two institutions for blind namely:-

(a) Technical Training Institute run by Poona Blind Men's Association, and

(b) The Poona School and Home for Blind Boys.

Though both the institutions are supposed to have 100 inmates each, but only 196 residents from these two institutions could be contacted, who formed the material for the study. The period of study was from 1 May to 31 October 1985.

A pretested schedule incorporating the findings of the interview, those of eye examination and the study of psychological aspects of each individual, were utilised for the study. The schedule was prepared in consultation with the Eye Specialist and Clinical psychologist of the Armed Forced Medical College, Pune.

For assessing the psychosocial profile of the study subjects, a Multiphasic Questionnaire (MPQ) was used as a scale.

Socioeconomic status of the subjects was assessed by using Kuppuswamy's scale (1976).

Findings and Discussion

Age and Sex Distribution

Age of the study population ranged from 6 to 40 years with

male : female ratio of 13 : 1. Two thirds of the subjects were aged less than 20 years. However, the age distribution in the present study may not be representative of that of the general population. Sharma and Prasad (1962) in their epidemiological study reported maximum blindness in the age group of 60-65 years. Similarly, Srivastave and Verma (1978), Chakrabarti et al (1974) and Gupta et at (1983) also observed higher proportion of blindness in the older age groups.

In various surveys a higher prevalence of blindness was found among female population, which was attributed to higher incidence of trachoma, conjuctivitis and cataract among them (Roy, 1984). The preponderence of male subjects in the present study may be attributed to the fact that out of the two institutions, one was entirely for boys and the other had only 14 female subjects out of 97 individuals examined. This probably could part of parents of female children to send their blind daughters away from home for any vocational education and training.

Educational Status

The relationship between literacy status and blindness is shown in table 1.

Table 1

Distribution of the study population by education

	Illiterate	*Primary School*	*Middle School*	*High School*	*Hr. Sec*	*Graduate & above*	*Total*
Number	25	91	33	43	3	1	196
Percentage	12.75	46.43	16.84	21.94	1.53	0.51	100.0

Table 1 shows that about 87 percent of study population was literate, 22.98 percent had education beyond high school.

Studies by Bhalerao (1983) and Batra (1981) also comprised of higher proportion of literate blind subjects. Both the present one and other studies cited above, do not represent true literacy status among the blind in general population.

Distribution by Social Class

Table 2

Distribution of study population according to social class

Social class	*Number*	*Percentage*
I	3	1.53
II	20	10.20
III	43	21.94
IV	129	65.82
V	1	0.51
Total	196	100.00

Table 2 shows that two-thirds of the study subjects were from lower social class and there was a gradual increase in proportion of study population with lowering of social status.

In is a well established fact that people from lower socio-economic status have higher prevalence of blindness. Sharma and Prasad (loc cit) and Mehta (1977) in their studies of the institutionalised blind also reported higher proportion of subjects among lower socio-economic status.

Acceptance of the Blind by Other Members of the Family

Table 3

Acceptance of the blind by members of the family

	Parents		*Spouse*		*Children*		*Others*	
Acceptance	*Number*	*Percentage*	*Number*	*Percentage*	*Number*	*Percentage*	*Number*	*Percentage*
Yes	149	90.30	24	80.00	11	100.00	139	87.42
No	16	9.70	6	20.00	-	-	20	12.58
Total	165	100.00	30	100.00	11	100.00	159	100.00

Table 3 depicts that most of the relatives showed due concern and affection and also accepted the blind as members of the family. Majority of the study subjects were not neglected by their relatives. Findings of the present study are similar to those of Bhalerao (loc cit) and Batra (loc cit).

Reaction of Strangers

About 91 percent of the blind subjects felt that their friends were helpful, had accepted them with respect and mingled freely with them. 97.45 percent subjects also expressed that even the strangers behaved with sympathy and understanding. The findings of the present study are in confirmity with those of Bhalerao (loc cit).

Invitation to Social Functions

About 92 percent of the study subjects were invited to various social functions and gatherings by their relatives and friends. The findings of the present study could be compared favourably with those of Bhalerao (1983) where also majority of the cases were invited to household functions and even neighbours helped in escorting them to various public/social functions.

Blindness and Marital Life

Out of 30 married subjects of the study population, about 80 percent confirmed that they experienced contentment in their married life. Further analysis revealed that there was no association between contentment in marital life and literacy and social status or with the scale of sightedness of the spouse.

Attidute of the people towards life

About 52 percent of the study population, most of them being children and adolescents aged between 6 and 18 years, were optimistic about their future. They did not feel deterred by their disability and hoped to do well in the future life. About 47 percent of the subjects were neutral in their attitude towards life and were fatalistic They had taken the disability in their own stride.

Psychological Aspects

Only about 19 percent of the study subjects showed valid results to psychological scoring by multiphasic Questionnaire (MPQ) and the results are shown in table 4 below.

Table 4

Distribution of the subjects showing valid tests to MPQ

	Normal	*Abnormal*	*Total*
Number	23	14	37
Percentage	62.16	37.84	100.00

It is evident from the above table that about 62 percent of the blind subjects showed normal personality profile and 38 percent with one or more abnormal traits.

Various psychological traits seen among subjects with abnormal protile were analysed further and are shown in table 5.

Table 5

Abnormal psychological profile

Psychological traits	*Number of subjects*	*Percentage*
Manic	11	29.73
Depressive	6	16.22
Hysterical	5	13.51
	4	10.81
	1	2.70
Schizoid	-	-
Anxiety	-	-
Psychopathic deviate	-	-
Total	27	

Note: Total number of subjects (27) in the above table is more than the number of subjects showing abnormal personality proñle (14) because few of the subjects showed more than one abnormal trait.

Main abnormal traits shown were mania, depression, hysteria and paranoid. Only one individual showed schizoid state.

The blind go through phases of disbelief, protest, depression and final recovery.

Bansal et al (1980) studied six areas of psychological aspects among visually impaired and found significantly high score in the area of depression and tension. Checkley and Slade (1979) reported a case of schizophrenia in a blind individual. These findings are consistent with those of the present study except for the manic aspects seen among some of the blind subjects. This could be explained to defence mechanism to conceal their depression.

One thing noteworthy was that none of the study subjects showing valid results to MPQ presented anxiety, contrary to expectation, in their personality profile. Confidence gained by the subjects under study and absence of anxiety were probably due to education, vocational training and also because they were in their own crowd.

In conclusion, it may be said that the institutionalised blind people in the study population were probably more accepted by their own family members as well as by the strangers. Most of the study subjects were found to be quite optimistic about their future life. But still about 38 percent showed one or more abnormal psychological traits. Abnormal personality profile in 38 percent of the study population was pretty high compared to 10.2 percent psychiatric morbidity among rural and 2.39 percent in urban population respectively as reported in various psychiatric field studies in India (Shah, 1984).

The present study indicated that periodical psychological assessment and psychotherapy should form the management of the blind which has been neglected hitherto.

Summary

A psychosocial study of 196 institutionalised blind individuals was carried out for a period of six months. Age, sex, educational and social status of the study population have been discussed. Acceptance of blind subjects by their family members, friends and strangers and their attitude towards life and their abnormal psychosocial profile have been highlighted in this communication.

Reference

1. Bansal RK, Jain IS, Kohli TK, Bansal SL, Psychological factors associated with visual impariment.

   Indian J. Psychiatry, 1980, 22, 173-5.

2. Batra Sushma. Social Integration of the Blind. New Delhi, Naurang, 1981.

3. Bhalerao Usha. Educated Blind of Urban Madhya Pradesh (A Sociological Study). New Delhi, Sterling Publishers Pvt Ltd 1983' 19-24.

4. Chakraborti, J. Garg AC. Sidha CMS. Prevalence and pattern of blindness in field practice area of rural health training centre. Indian J. Ophthalmology, 1974, 22, 4; 4-8.

5. Checkley SA, Slade AP. Bindness and Schizophrenia (letter) Lancet, 1979, 1(8118), 730-1.

6. Khurana AK, Saikia KL, Parmar PS, Aggarwal SKC. world Health Organisation. The prevention of blindness-Report of a WHO Study Group.

   WHO Tech Rep Ser No. 518, 1973.

7. Kuppuswamy B. Manual of Socio-economic status status scale, Manasayam, 32 Netaji Subhash Marg, Delhi.

8. Mehta DS. Hand Book of Disabled in India. Madras, Allied Publishers Private Ltd, 1983, 51-2.

9. Mehta Shashi. A study of the institutionalised blind in Maharashtra. A dissertation submitted for MS (Ophthalmology), University of Poona, 1977 (unpublished).

10 Park JE, Park K. Text Book of Preventive and Social Medicine, 10th edn. Jabalpur, M/S Banarsidas Bhanot, 1985.

11. Roy IS. Changing pattern of blindness in India. Indian J. Pub Heth 1984, 28, 221-6.

12. Shah VD. Mental Health Services in India. Psychiatry in India, First edn. Bombay, Bhalani Book Depot, 1984; 733-56.

13. Sharma KL, Prasad BG. An epidemlogical study of Blindness in Banki Block of Barabanki District (U.P.).

    Indian J. Med Res. 1962, 50; 842-65.

14. Srivastava RN, Verma Bl. An epidemiological study of blindness in an Indian rural community, J. Epidemiology and Community Health, 1978, 32; 131-5.

SECTION III

FAMILY PLANNING & MCH

Chapter–7

A Medico Social Study of 'MR' Acceptors

Introduction

Menstrual regulation, popularly known as 'MR' procedure is one of the most promising earlly postconceptional contraceptive mcthods which is now being widely used all over the world as a supplementary meaure of fertility control. Kessel and associates[5] defined 'MR' as treatment of delayed menstrual period within 13 days of the expected onset of menstrual cycle to ensure that a woman is not pregnant and does not remain pregnant". This method of fertility control is moving rapidly into the present gap between 'foresight contraception' and 'hindsight abortion' with additional risks[9]. This procedure involves vacuum aspiration of the uterine cavity within two weeks after last menstrual period. The rationale for the MR technique as most experts agree, is based not only on demographic, medical or legal arguments, but also on human needs. Concept of MR as a measure for fertility control is of recent one and promises to play a vital role in the National Family Planning Programme for effective fertility control in the future.[9, 10]

Keeping in view that MR procedure is an effective fertility control measures in early pregnancy, an attempt was made to ascertain various medico-social aspects among the acceptors attending a MR clinic in a military hospital.

Materials and Methods

All 318 women, who attended MR clinic of Command

Hospital, Pune between January 1982 and December 1983 formed the study population. Detailed information on various medico-social aspects of the acceptors e.g. age, religion, socio-economic, literacy and pregnancy status inlcuding acceptance of family planning methods following MR precedure and complications, if any, were collected from MR clinic, attached with Post Partum Cell of Armed Forces Medical College (AFMC).

Results

Majority of the acceptors i.e. 77.3% of women were in age group of 20-29 years, whereas 17% were in 30-45 yeara age group. Only 5.7% belonged to 15-19 years.

Out of 318 study subjects who underwent MR procedure, majority (86.9%) were Hindu and remaining (13.1%) were Muslims, Christains and Sikhs.

Table 1 revealed that 79.2% of acceptors were educated upto secondary school and above, while 10.4% were educated upto primary and only 9.7% were illiterate.

Table 1

Distribution of MR acceptors according to educational status

Education	*Number of acceptors*	*Percentage*
Illiterate	31	9.7
Primary	33	10.4
Secondary	131	41.3
Higher Secondary	51	16.0
University	72	22.6
Total	318	100.0

The destribution of MR acceptors according to Kuppuswamy's classification for socio economic status scale, revealed that majority (45.9%) belonged to social class III, followed by class I (25.2%) and class II (17.6%). Only 11.3% of acceptors were from class IV.

Table 2

Socio-economic status of the study population

Socio-economic Class	*Number of acceptors*	*Percentage*
I	80	25.2
II	56	17.6
III	146	45.9
IV	36	11.3
V	-	-
Total	318	100.0

96.4% of the acceptors were married, while 1.55 were unmarried and 2.1% were living separated.

Majority of women (68.5%) were having one or two children whereas 26.8% were having 3 or more children. Only 4.7% of acceptors had no living child. (Table 3).

Table 3

Distribution of accepters according to the number of living children

Number of living children	*Number of accepters*	*Percentage*
Nil	15	4.7
1	107	33.6
2	111	34.9
3	66	20.8
3 or above	19	6.0
Total	318	100.00

It was observed from table 4 that pregnancy status was confirmed only amongst 73.3% of the acceptors. The percentage of confirmation rose from 56.9% to 78.1% with increase from 5 to 6 weeks of amenorrhoea. The rise in the proportion of confirmed cases was statistically significant. ($p < 0.01$).

Table 4

MR acceptors according to the period of gestation

Duration of amenorrhoe	*Number of women*	*Percentage*	*Pregnancy confirmed*	*Per-centage*
Upto 5 weeks	72	22.6	41	56.9
Upto 6 weeks	246	77.4	192	78.1
	318	100.0	233	73.2

$X^2 = 12.7$ df = 1 P < 0.01

Pregnancies were confirmed in 233 (73.2%) cases after histopathological examination while rest 85 (26.8%) cases showed endometrium with varied form of ovarian activities. Adenomatous hyperplasia was present in 4 (1.2%) cases and endometrial tuberculosis was in 2(0.9%) cases. (Table 5).

Only 7 cases (2.1%) had develolped some minor complications viz., mild pain, nausea, menstruation like discomfort and spotting either during or following MR procedure.

Table 5

Endometrial profile of non-pregnant cases with MR

Endometrium	*Number*	*Percentage*
Proliferative	32	10.1
Secretory	140	4.4
Mixed	11	3.4
Cystic glandular hyperplasia	22	6.9
Adenomatous hyperplasia	4	1.2
Endometrial tuberculosis	2	0.9
Total	85	26.8

From table 6 it is revealed that amongst MR acceptors, 134 (42.2%) cases did not use any contraceptive devices preceeding MR precedure. Furthermore, concomittant with MR procedure, 126(39.6%) cases accepted IUD insertion and 59(18.5%) cases underwent tubectomy operations.

Table 6

Distribution of contraceptive methods used by the acceptors before and after MR procedure

Method	*Before MR*		*After MR*	
	Number	*Percentage*	*Number*	*Percentage*
Tubectomy	-	-	59	18.5
Vasectomy	-	-	26	8. 2
IUD	7	2.1	126	39.6
Oral Pills	13	4.2	36	11.3
Condoms	148	46.5	59	18.6
Withdrawal methods	16	5.0	-	-
No methods	134	42.2	12	3.8
Total	318	100.0	318	100.0

Discussion

In the present study comprising 319 women, 77.3% accepters belonged to age group 20-29 years. This finding is in conformity with those of Kanitkar[4] (i.e. 77.1%) and Brenner et al[2] (ie 83.2%). However the percentage was found to be comparatively less (63.8%) by Mullick and Dawn[8]. The relatively high proportion of acceptors found in this age group of 20-29 years could be attributed to this being the most fertile period during a woman's reproductive life.

In the present series 86.9% were Hindus and 13.1% of women were from other religions e.g. Muslims, Christians and Sikhs. These observations compare favourably with findings of Annual Family Planning Year Book[3].

In this study, the educational level of acceptors with secondary and above was appreciably higher (79.8%) as compared to the findings of Kanitkar and Walvekar[1] (ie 72.0%). However, Mullick and Dawn[8] in another study found that 65.4% of the MR acceptors were illiterate or with primary educational level.

In the present study, there was encouraging response from women belonging to socio-economic class III (45.9%) followed by I and II (42.8%). Most of the acceptors were found to be of moderately higher socio-economic class. However, Khandwala and Pai[6] reported that 90.5% cases were having income more than Rs. 300.00 per month.

In this series, 96.4% of women were married, which is in conformity with the findings (99.15) of Mullick and Dawn[8].

Majority of the acceptors (89.3%) had 1 to 3 living children. The women came for MR procedure mostly due to spacing, limitation of family size and socio-economic reasons. The present study indicated a comparatively higher proportion of cases in contrast to Mullick and Dawn[8] reporting 46.3% in their series. The higher percentage in this study could be due to increased awareness among families of Defence services who are regular and permanent beneficiaries of chain of family welfare centres in various military garrisons.

In the current series, the confirmation of overall pregnancy status was established among 73.3% of acceptors. 56.9% were confirmed within first week after missed menstrual period, whereas 78.1% after the second week and the difference was highly significant ($p < 0.01$). But Kanitkar and Walvekar[4] observed 70 and 27% of the acceptors reporting of MR after one week and between 10 to 15 days respectively in their series.

In the present study, histopathological examination of endometrial tissues among 85 (26.9%) non-pregnant cases revealed varied form of ovarian activities. Proliferative endometrium was observed in 10.1% of the cases followed by secretory phase (4.4%), 2 cases of endometrial tuberculosis were also detected. In the series reported by Kanitkar and Walvekar[4], the respective percentage of endometriosis were found to be as 14 and 28% with prolifeative and secretory changes in the endometrium. There was only one case of TB endometriosis in their study.

The incidence of complications after MR is an important parameter for evaluating the safety of the procedure. In the current series, only 7 cases (2.1%) had developed minor complications like mild pain, cramp, nausea, menstruation like discomfort and spotting whereas Agarwal and Kinra[1] in their series observed that 10% of the cases had reported with minor symptoms.

Acceptance of contraceptives is one of the important factors to make impact on the family planning programme. In the present series, 42.2% did not adopt any contraceptive device before undergoing MR. However 26.7% of the acceptors and their spouses were motivated to undergo sterilisation operations along with appreciable increase of 16.7% in adoption of any of the temporary methods. The increase in percentage of IUD acceptors after the procedure was found to be 37.5% which is much higher than the finding i.e. 20.0% as reported by Agarwal and Kinra.[1]

Summary

A medico-social study was carried out among 318 women seeking menstrual regulation (MR) procedure at Command Hospital (Southern Command) Pune between January 1982 and December 1983. All acceptors wanted to avoid undesirable early pregnancies. Various medicosocial aspects of the acceptors, namely age, religion, socio-economic and literacy status, number of living children, complication rates following the procedure etc. have been discussed. 95.5% subjects accepted contraceptive methods after MR. The procedure was found to be popular and acceptable. Endometrial profile of nonpregnant cases following MR were also analysed.

Menstrual regulation is recommended as a useful and effective addition to present fertility control methods in National Family Programme, being a simple, safe, effective and economic procedure.

Reference

1. Agarwal A. and Kinra G. : Menstrual Regulation. J. Obst and Gynae, India, 29, 2, 285-288, 1979.

2. Brenner FT.; Edelman, David A and Kessel E : Menstrual regulation in the United States: A Preliminary Report-Fertility and Sterility Vol 26, 209-295, 1975.

3. Family Welfare Programme in India. Year Book, 1975-76.

4. Kanitkar, SD, Walvekar, V. : Clinical experience with Menstrual Regulation (100 cases). J. Obst and Gynec. India, 25, 6 783-785, 1975.

5. Kessel, E. : A Menstrual Regulation in Family Planning Services. Published in Menstrual Regulation-A New Procedure for Fertility Control by CS Dawn, Ist ed. 125-136, 1975.

6. Khandwala, S.D. and Pai DN : Menstrual Regulation. J. Obst and Gynec India, 25, 6, 787-790, 1975.

7. Kuppuswamy, B. : Manual of Socio-economic status scale (Urban), Manasayan, 32 Netaji Subhash Marg, Delhi-6,1976.

8. Mullick B., Dawn CS. Menstral Regulation J. Obst and Gynec. India 25, 2 248-252, 1975.

9. Population Report-Menstrual Regulation : What is it? Series F, 2, 1973.

10. Population Report - Menstrual Regulation upto date series F, 4, 1974 Summary of 3 days Conference on Menstrual Rbulation-Sponsored by University of Hawaii, School of Public Health and School of Medicine held in H nolulu, Hawaii, 1973.

Chapter–8

Some Factors Associated with Decision Making among MTP Acceptors

Abstract

This study analyses the various factors associated with decision making for undergoing medical termination of pregnancy (MTP). The study was carried out among 88 women who had either undergone MTP or decided to undergo the procedure at Pune in two hospitals between April and September 1984. Associated factors like age of the acceptors, their social, marital and literacy status, number of living children and reasons for delay in decision making have been discussed.

Introduction

In order to curb the incidence of illegal abortions by quacks culminating them in high moriodity and mortality, the medical termination of pregnancy was declared legalised in our country since April 1, 1972 when the MTP Act, 1971 came into force.

When a woman wants to terminate an unwanted pregnancy various factors are involved in the decision making. The reasons for such a decision may include pregnancy before marriage or due to rape, incest or adultery or at times for fertility control either to limit family size or for spacing of children. Further, the reasons for fertility control may include her health, family income, unemployment, inadequate housing, interference with her education, training, etc.[1]

To be willing to interrupt her own pregnancy, a woman has to be highly motivated. Further, quicker the decision, better it is for the woman, to prevent the complications of abortion and its associated morbidity and mortality[2,3] The factors that can influence the promptness in decision making may be many and complex. Therefore, if these factors are known, MTP cannot only become technically easier but also safer, if done at earlier stages of pregnancy. Keeping these aspects in mind, the present study was undertaken to bring out the factors associated with the time interval between knowledge of pregnancy and decision to undergo medical termination of pregnancy.

Material and Methods

The study was carried out in Obstetrics and Gynaecology Out-patient Departments of Command Hospital, Pune and Sonawane Maternity Hospital, Pune during April-September, 1984. The study population comprised of 88 civilian women who had either already undergone MTP or decided to undergo the same.

The information was recorded on a schedule using personal interview technique. After establishing the initial rapport, the respondents were interviewed alone. During the interview, husband or relative was not permitted. At times, the help of local nurse or lady doctor was sought to bridge the communication gap in a few cases who knew only Marathi. By and large, it can be said that the respondents were frank and cooperative.

Findings and Discussion

Socio-demographic Characteristics of Respondents

The age distribution of respondents has been shown in Table 1. It is seen from this table that 65.91 per cent of respondents belonged to the age group 20-29 years. Similar findings have been reported by the authors of other studies[4, 5, 6]. A few other studies, however, mentioned that although the majority of cases belonged to 20-29 years of age group, but constituted about 55 per cent of total MTP cases[7, 8, 9]. Proportion of teenagers (11.36%) in the present study was higher than that reported by all India figures for MTP cases[5, 7]. Also, in the present study, three teenagers were less than 15 years of age and were not even in the conventional reproductive age group of 15-44 years.

Table 1

Distribution of respondents by age

Age in years	*Number*	*Percentage*
10-14	3	3.41
15-19	7	7.95
20-24	30	34.09
25-29	28	31.82
30-34	14	15.91
35-39	5	5.68
40 and above	1	1.14
Total	88	100.00

Out of 88 respondents, 76 (86.36%) were married and 8 (0.09%) unmarried. Widows and separated women constituted 3 (3.41%) and 1 (1.14%) of total respondents respectively. Similar findings have been reported in various other studies[9, 10, 11, 12, 13, 14]. Yet in another study, 6.9 per cent of MTP cases were reported of unmarried mothers while according to all India figures for MTP cases, 5.8 per cent were unmarried[14, 15]. However, some workers have reported that unmarried subjects constituted more than 10 per cent of total respondents[10, 12].

Decision Time and its Associated Factors

Promptness in taking the decision: Distribution of respondents according to time taken for making early/

delayed decision about MTP has been shown in Table 2. It is obvious from the table that majority of the respondents (70.45%) werew quick in taking an early decision (within a week's time after the confirmation of the pregnancy to go in for MTP. However, 26 respondents (29.55%) made a delayed decision (decision time of more than one week). Similar findings were also reported in other study in which 65% of respondents were made their decision to undergo MTP immediately on knowing about their pregnancy[16]. However, there was no mention of the time taken by the remaining 32 per cent. On the other hand, as per other study it was found that only 26.4 per cent made decision about MTP within one week.

Table 2

Distribution of respondents by Decision Time

Decision time (in weeks)	*Number*	*Percentage*
1	62	70.45
2	13	14.77
3	3	3.41
4	5	5.68
5	1	1.14
6 and above	4	4.55
Total	88	100.00

Decision maker for MTP: Distinction of respondents according to the decision maker has been given in Table 3. From the table, it can be noted that in majority of cases (38.64%), the decision was made mutually by the husband and wife. In case of 13 cases (14.77%), the decision was made by the respondents themselves and this group specifically included widows and separated women. For eight unmarried respondents (9.09%), the decision was made by the parents. However, in other study the husband was found to be the dominant decision maker (in 43.3% cases), followed by husband and wife mutually (32.6%)[10].

Table 3

Distribution of Respondents by Decision Maker

Decision maker for MTP	*Number*	*Percentage*
Husband	33	37.50
Self	13	14.77
Mutually by Husband and wife	34	38.64
Parents	8	9.09
Total	88	100.00

Age of respondents and decision making: The relationship between age of respondents and time taken for decision making has been shown in Table 4. It is evident from the table, that a higher percentage of teenagers (80%), made a delayed decision as compared to other age groups. The difference was found to be statistically significant.

Table 4

Decision Making According to Age of Respondents

Age in Years	*Decision Making*		*Total and*
	Early	*Delayed*	*Percentage*
10-14		3 (100.00%)	3 (100)
15-19	2 (28.57%)	5 (71.43%)	7 (100)
20-24	23 (76.67%)	7 (23.33%)	30 (100)
25-29	22 (78.57%)	6 (21.43%)	28 (100)
30-34	10 (71.43%)	4 (28.57%)	14 (100)
35-39	4 (80.00%	1 (20.00%)	5 (100)
40 and above	1 (100%)		1 (100)
Total	62 (70.45%)	26 (29.55%)	1 (100)

$X_2 = 5.62$ df = 1 $p < 0.05$

Marital status and decision making: Distribution of respondents according to their marital status and time taken for decision making has been presented in Table 5. It is seen from the table that a higher proportion of 'other man married' woman made a delayed decision as compared to the married ones. This difference is found to be statistically significant. Similar findings have also been reported by other researchers in their studies[6].

Table 5

Decision Making According to Marital Status of Respondents

Marital Status	*Decision Making*		*Total and*
	Early	*Delayed*	*Percentage*
Married	58 (76.32%)	18 (23.68%)	76 (100)
Unmarried	2 (25.00%)	6 (75.00%)	8 (100)
Widows	1 (33.33%)	2 (67.67%)	3 (100)
Separated	1 (100.00%)		1 (100)
Total	62 (70.45%)	26 (29.55%)	88 (100)

$X_2 = 7.25$ df = 1 $p < 0.01$

Table 6

Decision Making According to Religion of Respondents

Religion	*Decision Making*		*Total and*
	Early	*Delayed*	*Percentage*
Hindu	50 (68.49%)	23 (31.51%)	73 (100)
Muslim	5 (71.43%)	2 (28.57%)	7 (100)
Christian	3 (75.00%)	1 (25.00%)	4 (100)
Others	4 (100.00%)		4 (100)
Total	62 (70.45%)	26 (29.55%)	88 (100)

$X_2 = .34$ df = 1 $p < 0.05$

Religion and decision making: Table 6 clearly shows the relationship between religion of the respondents and the time taken for the decision making. It can be observed from the table that a higher percentage of Hindu women made a delayed decision as compared to non-Hindu women. However, this difference was not found to be statistically significant.

Occupation and decision making: The relationship between time taken for decision making and occupation of the respondents has been shown in Table 7. It is obvious that a higher percentage of housewives (34.38%) made a delayed decision as compared to others. This difference was, however, not statistically significant.

Table 7

Decision Making According to Occupation of Respondents

Occupation	*Decision Making*		*Total and*
	Early	*Delayed*	*Percentage*
Housewife	42 (65.62%)	22 (34.38%)	64 (100)
Service	11 (91.67%)	1 (8.33%)	12 (100)
Business	3 (100.00%)		3 (100)
Miscellaneous	6 (66.67%)	3 (3.33%)	9 (100)
Total	62 (70.45%)	26 (29.55%)	88 (100)

$X_2 = 2.63$ df = 1 $p < 0.05$

Educational status and decision making: The relationship between decision making time and educational status of the respondents has been presented in Table 8. The table shows that a greater proportion of illiterates (46.43%) made delayed decision as compared to literate individuals (21.6%). This difference was found to be statistically significant.

Table 8

Decision Making According to Educational Status

Education Status	*Decision Making*		*Total and*
	Early	*Delayed*	*Percentage*
Illiterate	15 (53.57%)	13 (46.43%)	28 (100)
Literate	47 (78.33%)	13 (21.67%)	60 (100)
Total	62 (70.45%)	26 (29.55%)	88 (100)

$X_2 = 5.62$ df = 1 $p < 0.05$

Social class and decision making: The relationship between decision making and social class of the respondents as per-Prasad's classification[17] has been shown in Table 9. It is evident from the table that a higher percentage and respondents belong to social class III and below made a delayed decisions compared to who were from social class I and II. The difference was found to be statistically significant.

Table 9

Decision Making According to Social Class

Social Class	*Decision Making*		*Total and*
	Early	*Delayed*	*Percentage*
I	14 (93.33%)	1 (6.67%)	15 (100)
II	24 (80.00%)	6 (20.00%)	30 (100)
III	16 (53.33%)	14 (46.67%)	30 (100)
IV	3 (50.00%)	3 (50.00%)	6 (100)
V	2 (100.00%)		2 (100)
Total	59 (71.08%)	24 (28.92%)	83 (100)

$X_2 = 8.54$ df = 1 $p < 0.005$

Table 10

Decision Making and Number of Living Children

No. of Living Chiildren	*Decision Making*		*Total and*
	Early *No. Percentage*	*Delayed* *No. Percentage*	*Percentage*
0		2 (100.00%)	2 (100)
1	10 (66.67%)	5 (33.33%)	15 (100)
2	25 (73.52%)	9 (26.48%)	34 (100)
3	18 (85.71%)	3 (14.29%)	21 (100)
4	4 (80.00%)	1 (20.00%)	5 (100)
5 and above	3 (100.00%)		3 (100)
Total	60 (75.00%)	20 (20.00%)	80 (100)

$X_2 = 4.69$ df = 1 $p < 0.05$

Number of living children and decision making: The relationship between number of living children and decision making time has been depicted in Table 10. It is obvious from the table that a higher percentage of subjects having two or less living children made a delayed decision as compared to those with three or more living children. This difference was found to be statistically significant.

Reasons for delay in decision making: On ascertaining from 26 respondents who made delayed decision for MTP, the reason for delay were found to be as under:

Ignorance of MTP facilies

Fear of disclosing pregnancy to parents specially in unmarried subjects

Preoccupation with other pressing household problems

Fear of surgical operations

Uncertainty about continuing the pregnancy

Contemplating married with consort

No specific reason

A WHO report almost similar reasons for delay in decision making has been reported[18].

Acknowledgement

The authors are grateful to the Senior Advisor in Obstetrics and Gynaecology, Command Hospital (Southern Command), Pune and the authorities of Sonawane Maternity Hospital, Bhawani Peth, Pune for according the permission and extending the necessary help in conducting this study.

References

1. World Healrth Organization (1970) Spontaneous and indced Abortion, *WHO Tech. Rep. Ser. No. 461.*
2. Roy. D. (1976) Family Planning Measures - Their Merits and Demerits, J. Indian Med. Assoc. 66, p. 265-268.

3. Konar, M., Lahiri, D., Saha, K. & Lahiri, D. (1973) Abortion Mortality (Ten Years Survey in Eden Hospital with critical analysis of last three years). *The Journal of Obstetrics & Gynaecology of India, 23.* p. 436-442.

4. Soni, D., Velankar, S. Kapoor, I. & Arvindakshan, T.K. (1976 Characteristics of Women Seeking Medical Termination of Pregnancy). *The Journal of Family Welfare,* XXII, p. 51-61.

5. Kanbargi, R. & Kanbargi, S. (1977) Some Aspects of Communication in Legal Abortions - A Case Study. *The Journal of Family Welfare.* XXX, p. 32-40.

6. Goraya, R., Mohan, D., Agarwal, N., Takkar, D., & Hingorani, V.A. Pilot (1975) Study of Demographic and Psycho-social Factors in Medical Termination of Pregnancy. *J. Indian Med. Assoc.* 64: p. 309-315.

7. Ministry of Health and Family Welfare. Family Welfare Programme in India Yearbook 1982-83. New Delhi, Ministry of Health and Family Welfare, Government of India.

8. Bose, C., & Sethna, N.J. (19) A Study on Induced Abortion in Married Women in an Urban Area. *The Journal of Family Welfare.* XXVI, p. 40-49.

9. Krishnamurti, N. & Manu, V. (1979) A Retrospective Study of the Demographic Characteristics of MTP Acceptors at a Postpartum Centre. *The Journal of Family Welfare.* XXVI: p. 30-40.

10. Singh, R. & Kashyap, P. (1980) Situational Variables of Women Seeking MTP at AIIMS Hospital, New Delhi, *Indian Journal of Preventive and Social Medicine.* 11: p. 124-129.

11. Rao, V.N. & Panse, G.A. (1975) Analysis of Acceptors of Medical Termination of Pregnancies in Maharashtra. *The Journal of Family Welfare.* XX, p. 64-73.

12. Kanitkar, S.D. & Rao, S.R. (1974) The Report of 150 Cases of Medical Termination of Pregnancy. *The Journal of Obstetrics and Gynaecology of India,* 24. p. 325-331.

13. Pandey, D.N., Agnihotri, S.P. Gupta K. & Kishore, N. (1979) An Analysis of Medical Termination of Pregnancies Performed during 1972. *The Journal of Family Welfare.* XXV: p. 41-45.

14. Ministry of Health Family Welfare. Family Welfare Programme in India Yearbook 1977-78. New Delhi Department of Family Welfare and Ministry of Family Welfare, Government of India.

15. Thakore, V.H., Shah. M. & Aggarwal, J.A. (1974) A Report on Medical Termination of Pregnancy in Gujarat, 1972-73. *The Journal of Family Welfare.* XX. p. 3-8.

16. Divekar, S.A., Natrajan, G. & Purandare, V.N. (1981) Report: MTPs - A Psychological Review. *Health and Population - Perspectives and Issues.* p. 199-211.

17. Prasad, B.G. (1970) Changes Proposed in the Social Classification of Indian Families. *Journal of Indian Medical Assoc.* 55. p. 198-199.

18. World Health Organization (1976) Induced Abortion. *WHO Tech. Rep. Ser. No. 623.*

Chapter–9

Socio-Demographic Profile of Tubectomy Acceptors

Abstract

An analytical study of the tubectomy acceptors was carried out in Army. About 85 per cent of volunteers were literate and had not used any contraceptive method earlier. More educational efforts should be undertaken to motivate the couple on the need to adopt contrapctive method, more so of terminal means after having two or more children.

Introduction

In India, the National Family Planning Programme was launched in 1952 and sterilisation, as a method of birth control, was officially introduced in 1956. This vital health programme was being promoted in the Armed Forces as a welfare measure long before it was introduced in the nationl programme. The sterilisation operation, especially tubectomy, has been found to be a very effective, dependable and one-time method to control the country's most formidable problem of population explosion. During 1985-86 alone, nearly 4.90 million sterilisation operations were performed in India and in the 7th Five Year Plan (1985-90) a target of 31 milllion sterilisation operations had been projected by the country's health planners and demographers.

Tubectomy constitutes the mainstay of the family planning programme of the armed forces. It is well known that a woman's motives for wanting to adopt terminal method of contraception are determined by her life situation as well as by the values and customs of the communicty in which she lives. A number of demographic and social variables play an important role in the acceptance of different contraceptive measures. For example, if a woman accepts the sterilisation operation after making her full contribution to the population situation, it becomes a sheer waste of national resources. Therefore, in order to promote the adoption of the terminal method after achieving the optimum family size, which in the national programme is the small family norm of two children, it is necessary to understand the socio-demographic factors associated with its acceptance.

Methodology

The present study was carried out in a few military garrisons during 1988. Secondary data, available with the seven Family Welfare Planning Centres (FWPC) (two class I and five class II) were collected using a pretested schedule with the help of staff of various health units through specialist officers and their staff. The data relating to all the 1124 tubectomy cases performed during 1987 was collected, collated and compiled from these FWPCs and statistically analysed.

Results and Discussion

Age at Acceptance

The distribution of respondents according their age at the time of tubectomy is presented in Table 1.

Table 1
Distribution by age at Sterilisation

Age at sterilisation (Years)	*No. of respondents*
15 - 19	1 (0.1)
20 - 24	235 (20.9)
25 - 29	496 (44.2)
30 - 34	301 (26.8)
35 - 39	88 (7.8)
40 - 44	2 (0.2)
Total	1123 (100.00)

Table 1 shows that as many as 65 percent of the respondents were in the age group of 20-29 years, and those under 20 constituted less than 1 percent.

Similar observations were made by Lila Ram et al in 1979, Jamshedji et al in 1980 and Yadav et al in 1984. However, in 1977, Mittal et al found maximum numbers of acceptors in the age group 30-34. National level figures for 1985-86 indicated 50 percent of acceptors in the 20-29 age group and about 31 percent in the 30-34 age group.

Further analysis of the data showed that the mean age of tubectomy acceptors in the present study was found to be 29.1. This was well below the mean age of sterilisation in India which was found to be 31.8 in 1986. Thus, it can be concluded that the spouses of army personnel in this study had accepted sterilisation at a comparatively younger age.

Religion

A religion-wise distribution indicated that the majority of the subjects (85.7 percent) were Hindu, followed by Sikhs (9.3%) and Muslims (3.1%) respectively; Christians constituted 1.9 percent of the sample.

Educational Status

The distribution of acceptors as per their educational status and that of their husbands is given in Table 2.

Table 2

Distribution of acceptors as per their educational status and that of their husbands

Literacy level	*Husbands*	*Acceptors*
Illiterate	140 (12.5)	158 (14.1)
Primary school	228 (20.3)	525 (46.7)
Middle school	222 (19.8)	191 (17.0)
High school	435 (38.7)	160 (14.2)
Graduate & above	98 (8.7)	89 (7.9)
Total	1123 (100.0)	1123 (100.0)

Figures in brackets denote percentages.

Table 2 shows that the majority of the respondents (46.7%) were educated upto the primary level and 39.2 percent were educated beyond this level. The proportion of illiterate respondents was low (14.1%) as compared to the findings of Shastri and Saha whose samples had 58.1 and 61.7 percent of illiterate acceptors respectively. The mean number of years spent in school was also found to be higher. The national figures among tubectomy acceptors indicated that almost half (49.5 percent) were illiterate, a third (33.4 percent) had completed upto primary school, and 10 percent upto middle school.

The literacy rate among sterilisation acceptors in the army was much higher as compared to the findings of other studies. The mean number of years spent in school was found to be 6.3 years which is higher than that of Lila Ram et al and Jamshedji et al, who reported durations of 4.6 and 4.5 years respectively, and far higher than those reported (2-3 years) by Yadav et al.

The literacy rate of the husbands of the acceptors was found to be higher -87.5 percent had received varying degrees of formal education with an average of 7-8 school years. This is comparable to the findings of other workers. At the all India level, as many as 40 percent of the acceptors and husbands were found to be illiterate, and about 37 and 12.5 percent had studied upto the primary and middle school levels respectively.

Rank-wise Distribution

A distribution of acceptors on the basis of the rank of their husbands revealed that 80.2 percent of the acceptors were wives of subordinate ranks other than officers or JCOs. There were 31 cases of tubectomy performed amongst the civilian defence employees (2.8 percent). The wives of officers and JCOs constituted 10.8 and 6.2 percent respectively of the sample.

Number of Children

The distribution of acceptors as per the number of children at the time of operation indicate that over half (51.6 percent) of the acceptors had three living children, about a third (31.4 percent) had two living children at the time of operation, and the rest (17%) had four or more children. Thus, about 83 percent of the respondents had three or fewer children at the time of tubectomy; at the national level, about 60 percent (1985-86) of the tubectomy acceptors had three or fewer living children. These findings are encouraging when compared to this and earlier studies which report that about 75 percent of the women had accepted sterilisation only after having four or more children, though Jamshedji et al had reported a slightly higher figure (55%).

The average number of children per acceptor was found to be 2.9. This compared favourably with the national average of 3.2. Earlier workers have observed averages ranging between 4.1 and 4.7.

Contraceptive Practice Prior to Sterilisation

Almost three-fifths of the acceptors (58.4%) had not used any contraceptive method prior to accepting sterilisation. Among those who had practiced contraception, the IUD was found to be the most popular method (15.7 percent acceptance) followed by Nirodh (11.9 percent acceptance). The oral pill was found to be least popular and had been used by 8.3 percent of the acceptors prior to adopting the terminal method, while about 5.6 percent mentioned the use of other conventional methods.

Khorana and others, also observed very low use of contraception among tubectomy acceptors prior to sterilisation acceptance. However, Sadasiviah reported that the IUD was used by 18.2 percent of his acceptor sample before switching over to tubectomy. The popularity of the IUD was not unexpected considering the wide publicity it had received and its easy availability at family welfare centres.

Conclusion

In conclusion, it may be mentioned that the maximum number of acceptors in this study were Hindus in the age group 20-29 years. Most of them (85.9 percent) were literate, had approximately three living children and about 60 percent had not used any contraceptive method earlier.

An in-depth evaluation of the programme needs to be carried out periodically so as to not only to consolidate the gains of health education achieved so far but also to motivate couples on the need for small families and the necessity for spacing births with non-terminal contraceptives.

References

1. Government of India, Ministry of Health and Family Welfare: Family Welfare Programme in India, Year Book 1986-87, Ministry of Health and Family Welfare, Department of Family Welfare, New Delhi.
2. Lilaram, D. and Basu, S.: Indian Journal of Gynecology & Obstetrics. 17:15-18 (1972).
3. Jamshedji, A. and Pachauic, S.: "The sterilisation decision - A socio-demographic and fertility profile of Indian women", The Journal of Family Welfare, 26(3) : 27-41 (1980).
4. Yadav, N.K. Singh, R.B. Mathews J.S: Indian Journal of Preventive and Social Medicine, 15 (1-2) : 27-29 (1984).
5. Mittal, M.C. Tiwari, S.C. and Patodi R.K. : Indian Journal of Public Health, 21 (2): 74-77 (1977).
6. Shastry, P.P.: "A demographic study of tubectomy acceptors of Ratnagiri district". The Journal of Family Welfare, 23 (2) : 90-96 (1976).
7. Saha. S.P.: Indian Journal of Public Health 26 (3): 117-128 (1981).
8. Verghese I. :"Tubectomy camps: A case study". The Journal of Family Welfare. 17 (4): 75-86 (1971).
9. Mehta, D.C. Shaw, N.H. and Khatri, T.D.: "Demographic characteristics of tubectomy acceptors in Kaira district". The Journal of Family Welfare 22 (1) 32-40 (1975).
10. Sadashivaiah, K. Ramesh A.S. and Sinha. J.S: "A comparative study of post-abortion sterilisation and general sterilisation". The Journal of Family Welfare, 23 (1) 21-26 (1976).
11. Khorana, A.B. :"Acceptor characteristics of women undergoing tubectomy". The Journal of Family Welfare. 22 (3) : 33-39 (1976).

Chapter–10

Utilisation of Health Services By High Risk Children Under Five in a Slum Area

Abstract

A cross sectional study was carried out to estimate the proportion of 'high risk' children under five in a slum area of Pune. The magnitude of the problem was considerable, the prevalence rate being 51.7 per cent. In this study, an attempt was also made to determine the extent of utilisation of available health facilities by this group, which was found to be 56.8 per cent. The association between utilisation of those facilities and various social factors like awareness, type of family, educational and occupational status of parents, socio-economic class etc. have been discussed.

Introduction

Children under five years of age constitute about 17 per cent of total population of India and 40 per cent of total annual deaths are contributed by this age group[1].

Children are most vulnerable group to diseases, disability and death. Certain proportion of the children are at special risk of diseases, its complications or death because of few factors in their biological make up, their environment or both. These 'risk factors' exert their effect singly or in combination[2].

The utilisation of health facilities is conditioned by number of interacting factors. Among these, type of family, social class and literacy status are of vital importance. Other equally significant determinants are distance involved from medical centre, attitude of professional rendering the service, quality of health needs and health awareness of the beneficiaries[3, 4, 5].

This community based study was undertaken to estimate the prevalence of 'high risk' children under five years of age at a point of time in a urban area of Pune. In this study attempts were also made to find out the extent of utilisation of health facilities by the parents of the 'high risk' children.

Material and Methods

A cross sectional survey was conducted for seven months in a slum area of Pune (New Modikhana). A complete coverage of all the children under five years was attempted through single home visits. However, due to non-availability of some of the occupants, 353 out of a total of 370 households could only be covered which comprised 340 children under five years of age. This constituted the material for the study. Relevant information in respect of each subject was collected in a pre-tested schedule.

Methodology adopted in this study for identifying 'high risk' child was based on the recommendations of WHO Expert Group and other workers[6, 7, 8, 9].

Medical and health facilities are provided to the community under study through Vallabh Bhai Patel Cantonment General Hospital, Pune which has 100 beds for inpatient treatment and also runs OPD in the hospital and 3 peripheral dispensaries. This hospital is situated about one kilometer away from New Modikhana. For specialised treatment, people of this area utilise Command Hospital (Southern Command) and BJ Medical College and Sassoon General Hospital, which are located about 3 to 6 kilometers away respectively. A few residents are covered under Central Government Health Scheme (CGHS) and Employees State Insurance (ESI) Scheme. There are two qualified medical practitioners within the locality and many more in the nearby areas.

Results

I. Prevalence of 'high risk' children

Out of 340 children under five years of age, 176 were identified as 'high risk' constituting a prevalence rate of 51.7 per cent, as shown in Table 1.

Table 1
Prevalence of 'High Risk' Children Under Five

Children under five	*'High risk' children*		*Not 'at risk'*	
	No.	Percentage	No.	Percentage
340	176	51.8	164	48.2

II. Utilisation of health facilities by parents of 'high risk' children and their sources

It was observed that out of 176 identified 'high risk' children, only 100 children (56.8 per cent) utilised available health facilities and rest 76 (43.2 per cent) did not make use of it. Parents of 40 per cent children 'at risk' utilised these facilities from Cantonment General Hospital, 30 per cent from Command Hospital (Southern Command), 10 per cent from qualified medical personnel and rest 20 per cent from other sources including ESI dispensaries, Medical College Hospital and Infectious Disease Hospital.

III. 'High risk' children and parents' awareness about risk factors

Parents numbering 76 of 'high risk' children who had not utilised any available health facility, were not also aware of presence of any 'risk factor' in their children. Out of the risk factors present though parents remaining unaware, were found to be having birth interval less than two years (40.8 per cent) followed by malnutrition (22.3 per cent), mother economically active (15.8 per cent) and birth order 5 or more (13.2 per cent). It was apparant that the nature of risk factors were such that it did not warrant the parents to seek health care as shown in Table 2.

Table 2

Distribution of 'High Risk' Children who were not utilising health facilities due to unawareness of 'Risk Factor'

S.No.	'Risk Factor'	'High risk' children unaware of 'risk factor'	
		No.	Percentage
1.	Birth interval less than two years	31	40.8
2.	Malnutrition-weight 70 per cent or below of 50th percentile of Harvard standard	17	22.4
3.	Birth order 5 or more	10	13.2
4.	Working mother and child looked after by a substitute	12	15.0
5.	Father being chronic alcoholic	6	7.0
	Total	76	100.00

Table 3

Distribution of 'High Risk' Children Under Five utilising health facilities by the type of family

Type of family	No. of 'high risk'	Health facilities utilised		Health facilities not utilised	
		No.	Percentage	No.	Percentage
Nuclear	65	27	41.5	38	56.5
Joint	111	73	65.8	38	34.2
Total	176	100	56.8	76	43.2

$X_2 = 9.80$; df=1; $p < 0.005$

IV. Utilisation of health facilities by type of family

'High risk' children from joint families (65.8 per cent) utilised health facilities more than those belonging to nuclear ones (41.5 per cent). The association between the utilisation and type of family was found to be highly significant ($p < 0.005$). This may be due to the fact that more members in the joint family could take care of 'high risk' children in utilising the existing facilities as in Table 3.

V. Utilisation of health facilities as per literacy status of father

Utilisation of health facilities increased with the rise in educational status of father is shown is Table 4. The association between utilisation of health facilities and literacy status of father was highly significant ($p < 0.001$).

Table 4

Distribution of 'High Risk' Children Under Five Utilising Health Facilities by Education of Father

Education of father	*No. of 'high risk'*	*Health facilities utilised*		*Health facilities not utilised*	
		No.	*Percentage*	*No.*	*Percentage*
Illiterate	32	7	21.9	25	78.1
Primary School/Literate	41	22	53.7	19	46.3
Middle	68	42	61.8	26	38.2
High School	28	23	82.1	5	17.9
Graduate	6	5	83.3	1	16.7
Postgraduate/ Professional	1	1	100	-	-
Total	176	100	56.8	76	43.2

X2 = 25.77; df=3; p<0.001

Note: Rows 4, 5 and 6 have been combined for statistical analysis.

VI. Utilisation of health facilities and education of mother

Utilisation of available health facilities was more among those 'high risk' children whose mothers were educated upto middle school and above and lower among those whose mothers were illiterate or had studies upto primary level. The association between utilisation of health facilities and education of mother was stastistically not significant ($p > 0.05$; as given in Table 5.

Table 5

Distribution of 'High Risk' Children Under Five Utilising Health Facilities by Education of Mother

Education of Mother	*No. of 'high risk'*	*Health facilities utilised*		*Health facilities not utilised*	
		No.	*Percentage*	*No.*	*Percentage*
Illiterate	46	28	60.9	18	39.1
Primary school/Literate	56	25	44.6	31	55
Middle	45	28	62.2	17	37.8
High School	27	17	62.9	10	37.0
Graduate	1	1	100.0	-	-
Postgraduate/ Professional	1	1	100.0	-	-
Total	176	100	56.8	76	43.2

X2 = 5.11; df= 3; p>0.05

Note: Rows 4, 5 and 6 have been pooled for statistical analysis.

VII. Utilisation of health facilities and occupation of father

It is seen from table 6 that utilisation of health facilities by 'high risk' children increased as the occupation of father improved. The association between utilisation of health facilities and occupation of father was highly significant ($p < 0.001$).

Table 6
Distribution of 'High Risk' Children Under Five Utilising Health Facilities by Occupation of Father

Occupation of Father	*No. of 'high risk'*	*Health facilities utilised*		*Health facilities not utilised*	
		No.	*Percentage*	*No.*	*Percentage*
Unemployed	12	4	33.3	8	66.7
Unskilled	42	15	35.7	27	64.3
Semiskilled	65	41	63.1	24	36.9
Skilled	18	14	77.9	4	22.2
Semi-professional	1	1	100.0	-	-
Total	176	100	56.8	76	43.2

X2 = 15.49; df=2; p<0.001

Note: Rows 4, 5 and 6 have been combined for statistical analysis.

Table 7
Distribution of 'High Risk' Children Utilising Health Facilities by Occupation of Mother

Occupation of Mother	*No. of 'high risk'*	*Health facilities utilised*		*Health facilities not utilised*	
		No.	*Percentage*	*No.*	*Percentage*
House-wife	148	84	56.8	64	43.2
Full-time janitorial	8	3	37.5	5	62.5
Part-time janitorial	5	2	40.0	3	60.0
Full-time agri./industry	6	4	66.7	2	33.3
Full-time clerical or professional	9	7	77.8	2	22.2
Total	176	100	56.8	76	43.2

X2 = 0.14; df=1; p>0.05

Note: Rows 2, 3, 4 and 5 have been combined for statistical analysis.

VIII. The Utilisation of health services and occupational status of mother

It is observed from Table 7 that out of 148 'high risk' children identified whose mothers were housewives, 84 (56.8 per cent) utilised the existing health facilities while 64 (43.2 per cent) did not do so. Among 'high risk' children where mothers were working, children of clinical or professional occupation utilised more health facilities than that of part time or full time janitorial occupation. However, the difference in utilisation of health facilities by occupation of mother was statistically not significant.

IX. Utilisation of health facilities by socio-economic class

Higher the social class, the greater was the utilisation of health services by 'high risk' children. However, the association was statistically not significant ($p>0.05$) as shown in Table 8.

Table 8

Distribution of 'High Risk' Children Utilising Health Facilities by Social Class

Social Class	*No. of 'high risk'*	*Health facilities utilised*		*Health facilities not utilised*	
		No.	*Percentage*	*No.*	*Percentage*
1	4	4	100.0	-	-
2	42	28	66.7	14	33.3
3	82	46	56.1	36	43.9
4	47	22	46.8	25	53.2
5	1	-	-	1	100.0
Total	176	100	56.8	76	43.2

$X_2 = 5.40$; df=2; $p > 0.05$

Discussion

In this study, 51.7 per cent children were identified as 'high risk'. Prevalence rate in a rural community of Maharashtra and in a semiurban population of Delhi were 19.8 and 63.5 per cent respectively[6, 10]. Prevalence rates of a rural community in Haryana were 89.4 and 51.7 per cent 'high risk' children under 3 and 6 years respectively. The differences in prevalence rate in various studies could be due to adoption of different set of risk factors, qualitative and quantitative differences in the samples surveyed and qualification of investigators in different studies.

Out of 176 'high risk' children, only 100 (56.8 per cent) utilised available health facilities. It has been observed that in 1982, the facilities were utilsied by 61.2 per cent children which is in conformity with the present series[3]. However, in this study the utilisation was done by 80.3 per cent 'high risk' children, which was much higher than the current series10.

It is observed from Table 2 that parents of 76 children who were 'at risk' did not utilise the existing facilities because they were not aware about presence of any of the risk factors like birth interval less than two years, malnutrition, economically active mothers etc. It has also been reported that parents of high risk children e.g. with birth interval less than 2 years (42.6 per cent), birth order 5 or more (27.8 per cent) etc. did not seek health facilities.

It has been revealed by Table 3 that 'high risk' children from joint families (65.8 per cent) utilised facilities more than those from nuclear families (41.5 per cent). The association between utilisation and type of family was highly significant. However, in other studies this aspect was not considered and hence could not be compared.

It is seen from Table 4 that utilisation of health facilities increased with rise in educational status of father of 'high risk' children. The association between utilisation of health facilities and education of father was highly significant ($p < 0.001$). Other studies also found significant increase in the utilisation of health facilities with improvement of father's literacy status.

In contrast, as seen in Table 5, the association between utilisation of health facilities and mother's educational level was statistically not significant. This finding is in contrast to other findings where it was observed that with rise in education of mother, the utilisation of health facilities also increased.

As seen from Table 6, the association between utilisation of health facilities and occupation of father was highly significant ($p < 0.001$). This could be because occupation of father had a direct effect on economic status, acquisition of education and better knowledge of child health care and purchasing power for medicine.

However, Table 7 shows that the difference in utilisation of health facilities by 'high risk' children according to occupational status of the mother was statistically not significant.

While analysing utilisation of health facilities by socioeconomic class (14) (vide Table 8) the association was not statistically significant ($p > 0.05$). In other studies the utilisation of health facilities was found to increase with improvement in socio-economic class.

References

1. Central Institute of Research and Training in Public Cooperation and Child Development (1975) *Perspective of the Child in India,* New Delhi.

2. World Health Organisation Expert Committee (1979) *'Risk Approach for Maternal and Child Health Care'* Offset publication 39, Geneva.

3. Mukherjee, A.C. (1982) Utilisation of Maternal and Child Health Services by Authorised Families provided by Armed Forces Family Welfare Centre in Pune Cantonment. A Dissertation for M.D. (PSM) Examination of University of Poona.

4. Anand, B. & Srinivase, D.K. (1972) Certain Dimensions of Child Health Care in an Urban Community. *Indian Journal of Medical Research,* 60, p. 1824-34.

5. Sapru, R. Chutani, C.S., Srivastva, A.B.L. (1975) Factors associated with utilisation of urban MCH/FP programme - A record study of one centre. *NIHAE Bulletin*, 8:3.

6. Shah, P.M., Janarkar, A.R., Bhole, V.S. (1976) Community, wide surveillance of "at risk" under five in need of special care. *Journal of Tropical Paediatrics,* 22: 2, 103-107.

7. Morley, D. (1973) Paediatrics priorities in the developing world. Ist ed. London, Butterworth & Co. Ltd.

8. Ghose, S. (1976) The Feeding and Care of Infants and Young Children. 2nd ed., New Delhi. Voluntary Health Association of India.

9. Walia, B.N.S., Shah, P.M., Shah, K. (1979) Practical Maternal and Child Health.

10. Kapil, U. (1980) A study of "high risk" mothers and children under five years in a semi urban community. A Thesis for M.D. (PSM) Examination of University of Delhi.

11. Bansal, S.M. (1979) Study of prevalence of sickness in children under 3 years of age, identifying the "risk factors" of a rural community of Haryana. A Thesis for M.D. (PSM) Examination of M.D. University of Rohtak.

12. Lal, S. (1981) At "Risk Factor" in Rural Area. Indian Journal of Paediatrics. 48, p. 605-609.

13. Kothari, U., Mukherjee, B., & Kanwar, K.K. (1980) Health Services Utilisation in Rural Area. *Indian Journal of Paediatrics,* 19:4.

14. Kuppuswamy, B. (1976) Manual of Socio-economic Status Scale (Urban). Manasayan, 32 Netaji Subhash Marg, Delhi-110006.

Chapter–11

Utilisation of Health Services by "High Risk" Pregnant Women in a Semi Urban Community

Abstract

A cross sectional study was undertaken to estimate the prevalence of "high risk"pregnant women in a semi-urban community for seven months in 1987. The magnitude of the problem was considerable, the prevalence rate being 44.65 per cent. In the present study an attempt was also made to ascertain the extent of utilisation of available health services facilities by this vulnerable group, which was found to be 73.24 per cent. The association between utilisation of those facilities and various social factors like age of study subjects, literacy status of these women and their husbands, socio-economic status, duration of pregnancy etc. alongwith the reasons for their non utilisation have been discussed in this communication.

Introduction

The maternal mortality has considerably doclined in developed countries due to overall improvement in socio-economic status and provision of efficient maternal and child health (MCH) services. (1) However, it is still very high in developing countries because of several factors such as financial constraint, lack of trained manpower and an effective organizational set up on the part of the Government and its underutilization due to illiteracy, ignorance and poor communication on the part of the large beneficiaries. (2) It is against this background that the WHO Task Force in 1978 evolved the concept of "Risk Approach" for improved MCH care as a managerial tool in order to ensure maximum utilisation of existing resources by those who need them most. (3)

Certian proportion of pregnant women are at special risk of diseases, its complications or death because of their biological make-up, their environment or both. These factors are called "Risk Factors" which exert their effect singly or in combination. Primigravidae, higher parity, too frequent pregnancies and that too at extremes of age, previous child loss are some of the universally recognized risk factors. Early recognition and timely intervention by existing MCH services in respect of these risk factors largely depend upon their proper utilization by the mothers at risk.

The present community based study was undertaken to estimate the prevalence of "high risk" pregnant women at a point of time in a semi urban community of Pune and also to find out the extent of utilization of existing health services by them.

Material and Methods

A cross sectional study was carried out in New Modikhana area, a semi urban locality of Pune during the period May to November 1987. A complete coverage of all the pregnant women with history of amenorrhoea of 12 weeks and more was attempted through single home visits. Out of a total of 1821 families residing in this area, 1754 (96.32%) could be contacted. A total of 183 married women furnished history of amenorrhoea. However, in 24 cases, the duration of amenorrhoea was of less than 12 weeks and the diagnosis of pregnancy could not be established by clinical examination. These 24 cases were not included in the study population, which comprised of 159 pregnant women only.

The methodology adopted to identify the "high risk" pregnant women in the present study was based on the recommendations of WHO Expert Group and other workers (3, 4, 5, 6, 7, 8, 9). The relevant information collected from each study subject was recorded on a pretested schedule.

Observations and Discussion:

Table I : Prevalence of "High Risk" pregnant women

No. of Pregnant women	*"High Risk" Factor identified in*		*No "risk factor" identified in*	
	No.	*%*	*No.*	*%*
159	71	44.65	88	55.35

Table I reveals that out of 159 pregnant women 71 (44.65%) were identified to have "high risk" factors. Kapil studied the pregnant women of Begumpura, a semi urban locality of South Delhi, and found prevalence of high risk factors in 27.58% of them (8) while Shanti Indra et al reported a prevalence of 42 percent amongst lying in cases at Eden Hospital in Calcutta. The difference in the findings of the present study with these studies can be attributed to adoption of different sets of "high risk" factors, qualitative and quantitative differences in the sample surveyed and qualifications of the interrogators in the respective studies.

Table II : Utilisation of health services by "High Risk" Pregnant Women

No. of High Risk Pregnant women	*Health Services utilised by*		*Health Service not utilised by*	
	No.	*%*	*No.*	*%*
71	52	73.24	19	26.76

Table II shows that out of 71 "high risk" pregnant women, 52 (73.24%) were utilising the health services facilities whereas 19 (26.76%) were not utilising the same. In the study by Kapil the extent of utilisation of health services was found to be 50 per cent.(8) The difference in extent of utilisation may be due to qualitative difference in literacy/health educational status and accessibility of these services at the two different places.

Table III : Utilisation of health services by "high risk" pregnant women according to their age

Age group	*No. of "High Risk" pregnant women*	*Health services utilised*	*Health services not utilised*
15-19	8(11.26)	7 (87.50)	1 (12.50)
20-14	32 (45.08)	25 (78.14)	7 (21.86)
25-29	23 (32.38)	16 (69.60)	7 (30.40)
30 and above	8 (11.26)	4 (50.00)	4 (50.00)
Total	71 (100.00)	52 (73.24)	19 (26.76)

X = 2.13; df = 1; p > 0.05

Note: Rows 1, 2 and 3, 4 have been clubbed together for the purpose of statistical analysis

Figures in parentheses indicate percentages

Table III shows an inverse relationship betwen the age and the extent of utilisation of health services by "high risk" pregnant women. The utilisation which was 87.50 percent in the age group below 20 years declined to 50 percent among pregnant women above 30 years of age. The difference in utilisation of health services by differ nt age groups was however not found to be statistically significant (p > 0.05). In his study in Delhi, Kapil did not study the association between maternal age and utilisation of health services. (8) Murali and Kataria associated the reason of less awareness about the importance of antenatal care among elderly pregnant women to low level of health services utilisation. (10) Kothari et al also reported health services utilisation to a higher extent by young women. (11)

It is evident from Table IV that utilisation of health services by high risk pregnant women was maximum (90.90%) by those with educational status of SSC and above followed by those educated upto middle standard (76.66%) , and illiterate subjects (65%). This difference was however, not found to be statistically significant (p > 0.05). Both Kapil and Mukerjee reported increases in extent of health services utilisation with the rise in literacy status (8, 12). Education creates an awareness of existing health services and its importance in health promotion, which in turn results in its better utilisation.

Table IV : Utilisation of health services by "high risk" pregnant women by their educational status

Edu. Status of "high risk" preg. women	*No. of "High Risk" pregnant women*	*Health services utilised*	*Health services not utilised*
Illiterate	20 (28 .17)	13 (65.00)	7 (35.00)
Primary	10 (14.08)	6 (60.00)	4 (40.00)
Middle	30 (42.46)	23 (76.68)	7 (23.33)
SSC and above	11 (15.49)	10 (90.90)	1 (9.10)
Total	71 (100.00)	52 (73.24)	19 (26.76)

X = 2.60; df = 1; p > 0.05

Note: Rows 1, 2 and 3, 4 have been clubbed together for the purpose of statistical analysis

Figures in parentheses indicate percentages

Table V: Utilisation of health services by "high risk" pregnant women by their educational status of husband

Eduucational Status of husband	*No. of "High Risk" pregnant women*	*Health services utilised*	*Health services not utilised*
Primary	7 (9.85)	4 (57.14)	3 (42.85)
Middle	25 (35.22)	18 (72.00)	7 (28.00)
SSC/Graduate	39 (54.93)	30 (76.93)	9 (23.07)

$X^2 = 0.599$; df = 1; p > 0.05

Note: Rows 1 and 2 have been clubbed together for the purpose of statistical analysis

Figures in parentheses indicate percentages

Table V reveals an increase in utilisation of health services with rise in educational status of husband, However, the difference in the extent of utilisation was not found to be statistically significant ($p > 0.005$). Kapil also found increase in utilisation of health services with increase in educational status of husband.(8)

The distribution of "high risk" pregnant women according to their socio-economic status based on Prasad's classification (13) is presented in Table VI.

Table VI: Utilisation of health services by "high risk" pregnant women by their socio-economic status

Socio-Economic Status	*No. of "High Risk" pregnant women*	*Health services utilised*	*Health services not utilised*
Class I	12 (16.90)	12 (100.00)	- (-)
Class II	32 (45.07)	23 (71.87)	9 (28.13)
Class III	27 (38.03)	17 (62.96)	10 (37.07)
Total	71 (100.00)	52 (73.24)	19 (26.76)

$X^2 = 2.34$; df = 1; $p > 0.05$

Note: Rows 1 and 2 have been clubbed together for the purpose of statistical analysis

Figures in parentheses indicate percentages

Table VII : Utilisation of health services by " high risk" pregnant women by duration of their pregnancy

Duration of Pregnancy	*No. of "High Risk" pregnant women*	*Health services utilised*	*Health services not utilised*
3-6 months (2nd trimester)	40 (56.33)	26 (65.00)	14 (35.00)
7 months and above	31 (43.67)	26 (83.87)	5 (16.13)
Total	71 (100.00)	52 (73.24)	19 (26.76)

$X = 3.17$; df = 1; $p > 0.05$

Figures in parentheses indicate percentages

It is evident from Table VI that "high risk" pregnant women from socio-economic class I were utilising health services to the fullest extent (100%), followed by socio-economic class II (71.87) and then class III (62.96%). The difference in utilisation was, however not statistically significant ($p > 0.05$). Both Kapil and Mukherjee also reported an increase in utilisation of health services with increase in percapita income and socio-economic class respectively (8, 12).

Table VII shows that there was higher utilisation of health services during third trimester (7 months and above) of pregnancy (83.87%) as compared to second trimester of pregnancy (65%). Murali and Kataria in their study found that reason for late utilisation of health services was to ensure prompt help and treatment during confinement. (10)

Table VII: Utilisation of health services by "high risk" pregnant women by source of utilisation (n=52)

Source of utilisation	*"High Risk" pregnant women utilising Health Services*	
	Number	*Percentage*
Service Hospital	44	84.61
Family Welfare Centre	8	15.39
Total	52	100.00

Table VIII shows that majority of the "high risk" pregnant women (84.61%) were utilising health services provided by local Military hospital affiliated to Armed Forces Medical College, Pune, located at a distance of about 4 km from the area of study. Health services provided by the family welfare centre located in Cantonment General Hospital within a distance of 1 km were being utilised by 15.39% of the study subjects only. The utilisation of health services depends on the quality of services being provided, even, when an alternative source is available. This could be the reason for higher utilisation of services from the Military Hospital where specialist care in other fields of medical science is also readily available. Other workers did not include this aspect of relative preference for a source in their studies.

Table IX: Non utilisation of health services by "high risk" pregnant women by reasons for their non-utilisation

Reasons for non-utilisation	*No. of 'High risk" pregnant women*	*Percentage*
Recent arrival in area of study and ignorance of utilising health facilities	12	63.15
No complications or symptoms in current pregnancy	4	21.05
Unsuitable timing of sources	2	10.54
Long distance of source	1	5.26
Total	19	100.00

Table IX shows that recent arrival in the area of study and ignorance about existing health facilities was the main reason given by 63.15% cases, followed by 21.05% who did not feel the necessity for utilising the health services as they felt free from complications/symptoms. Only 2 cases (10.54%) mentioned about unsuitable timing and a lone case (5.26%) about long distance involved to the source as the reasons for non-utilisation. Available studies of other workers did not include this aspect.

Table X: Non utilisation of health services by "high risk" pregnant women with "risk factor" present

Reasons for non-utilisation	*No. of 'High risk" pregnant women*	*No. of 'High risk' preg. women not utilising services*
Anemia (Hb < 10 gm%)	22	7(31.81)
Time since last delivery less than 2 years	32	9 (28.12)
Past history of foetal/child loss	20	5 (25.00)
Pregnancy with systemic disease	4	1 (25.00)
Maternal age < 18 years	4	1 (25.00)
Maternal age < 35 years	5	1 (20.00)

Figures in parentheses indicate percentages.

Total exceeded 19 as some of the 'high risk' cases had more than one 'risk factor'.

Table X shows that anaemia with Hb level of less than 10 gm% was the commonest risk factor (31.81%) in pregnant women who did not avail the existing health services available followed by those who delivered less than 2 years earlier than previous delivery (28.12%), pregnancy with systemic disease (25%), maternal age less than 18 years (25%) and maternal age above 35 years (20%). These findings could not be compared with the available studies of other workers who did not include this aspect in their studies.

Conclusion and Recommendations:

The present study revealed that the proportion of "high risk" mothers was quite high (44.65%). The study also revealed that overall utilisation of existing health care services by "high risk" pregnant women was 73.24 per cent. Thus 26.76 per cent of these women did not utilise these services for various reasons, the commonest reason being recent arrival in the locality and ignorance about sources of availability of these services followed by inconvenient timings and distance involved. The study thus clearly brought out the necessity of regular domiciliary visits by concerned health staff, particularly for recently arrived, families for imparting proper health education and detailed information on existing health care facilities.

References:

1. World Health Organisation - World Health Statistics Annual 1981.
2. World Helath Organisation - Sixth Report on World Health Situation Part II, 1980.
3. World Health Organisation - Risk Approach for Maternal and Child Health Care. WHO offect publication No. 39,1978.
4. Dey DR. Role of Grand Multiparity in causation of High Risk Pregnancy. Journal of Obst Gyne India, 1977; 17:706-8.
5. Blair D. Social Factors in Obstetrics. Lancet 1949; 18: 1079-83.
6. Butlar NR. Bonham DG. Perinatal mortalty. Edinburgh and London, London E & S Livingstone Ltd. 1963.

7. Cliffer H. High risk pregnancy. N. Engl. J Med. 1964. 271:243-9.
8. Kapil U.A study of high risk mothers and children under five years in a semi urban community. A thesis for MD Preventive & Social Medical examination of University of Delhi 1980.
9. Shanti I., Roy N.N, Mukherjee K, Sarker R. Chatterjee S. Perinatal Mortality in high risk pregnancy. J. Obstet Gynecol India 1977; 27 : 699-705.
10. Murali I, Kataria KM. Perception regarding need for antenatal care among rural and urban women in Delhi. Indian J. Pub. Heth 1980; 24:68-75.
11. Kothari U. Mukherjee B, Kanwar K. Health services utilisation in rural area. Indian Paediatrics 1980 ; 19: 4-6
12. Mukherjee AC. Utilisation of maternal and child health services by the authorised families provided by Armed Forces Family Welfare Centre in Pune Cantonment. A disscrtation for MD (Branch V) Preventive and Social Medicine examination of University of Poona, December 1992.
13. Prasad BG. Changes proposed in Social classification of Indian famil.es J. Indian Med Assn. 1970; 55: 198-9.

SECTION IV
HEALTH EDUCATION

Chapter–12

Smoking and Its Hazards – What One Should Know

Abstract

Nicotine is revengeful to everybody irrespective of the form in which tobacco is smoked, be it cigarette, bidi, hookkah, chillum, cigar or pipe. If pays no heed to the appeal that the individual is only a mild or moderate smoker and not a heavy smoker. All smokers are exposed to potential health hazards.

Introduction

Love Lady Nicotine risks your life. Today, it is known that smoking is probably the largest single preventable cause of ill-health in the world. The epidemic of smoking related diseases is of such magnitude as to rival only infectious diseases or malnutrition as a public health problem in developing countries. The findings of the Royal College of Physicians mention that one in three cigarette smokers dies prematurely as a result of cigarette smoking and that, on an average, each cigarette smoked shortons thc lifc of the smoker by five-and-a-half minutes. It has been estimated that, in the world as a whole cigarette smoking is responsible for more than 1 million premature deaths each year. Statistics show that 90 per cent of all lung cancer deaths, 25 percent of deaths from cardiovascular diseases and 75 percent of all deaths from chronic bronchitis stem directly from smoking. Perhaps 10 porcent of all deaths among smokers are attributable to this habit.

The studies in India shown that the lung cancer risk for cigarette smokers is nearly nine times more than for non-smokers. Japan and the USA record relatively low incidence of lung cancer despite high cigarette consumption-one reason may be these smokers discard larger cigarette ends. Cigarette smokers in the UK and possibly in India, are three times more likely to suffer from chronic bronchitis than non-smokers. It has also been observed that the intensity of smoking was more important than its duration. A study in the UK, shows that those with chronic bronchitis run a higher risk of developing lung cancer. Cigarette smokers are also more than twice as likely to develop coronary heart disease and three times more likely to develop myocardial infarction than non-smokers. The relation between cigarette smoking and cerebro-vascular disease (stroke) is largely confined to the younger age groups; there is less effect after the age of 65 years. In young people, ischaemic diseases of the legs (Thrombo-angitis obliterans) appears to be confined almost exclusively to those who smoke.

Besides, the love for lady Nicotine is also associated with some more miseries such as development of cirrhosis of the liver and cancer of lip, oral cavity, pharynx, nose, larynx, trachea, oesophagus, urinary bladder, kidney and pancreas. Incidence of gastroduodenal ulcers has been found twice as high in smokers than in non-smokers. Smoking may increase mortality by delayed healing of ulcer. Smoking may affect expectant mothers by way of retarded foetal growth and increase in the risk of perinatal death.

Besides nicotine, mother tobacco has got another daughter also-isoprenoids and a son-the tar. However, nicotine is better known and more notorious because of its strong pharmacological actions. These actions include (i) vaso-constriction (narrowing of blood vessels), tachycardia (increased heart rate) and elevation of blood pressure, (ii) initial stimulation of salivary and bronchial secretion followed by inhibition (iii) excitation of respiration, vomitting, anti-diuretic actions, (iv) inhibition of stomach contractions and gastric secretions, delaying the emptying time of the stomach, (v) inhibition of appetite and reduction in body weight by some process over and above the effect on appetite, (vi) increased bowl activity and diarrhoea followed by decreased activity, (vii) release of epinephrine from adrenal medulla and 11-hydroxy-corticosteroids from the adrenal cortex, and (viii) increase in serum free fatty acids and triglycerides. Tar is a well-known carcinogen.

Smoking affects non-smokers too

Lady Nicotine is revengeful to everybody irrespective of the form in which mother tobacco is smoked-be it cigarette, bidi, hookkah, chillum, cigar or pipe. She pays no heed to the appeal that the individual is only a mild or moderate smoker and not a heavy smoker. All smokers are thus exposed to the potential health hazards inherent in smoking-the severity of effect being merely a question of intensity and duration of smoking. Lady Nicotine not only inflicts vengeance upon smokers but doesn't spare the company also which they keep, although such company may consist of non-smokers only. These non-smokers who inadvertently inhale the smoke generated by their smoker friends come in the category of 'passive smokers' 'involuntary smokers' or 'secondary smokers'. Apart from discomfort, such exposure may cause distress to asthmatics and other susceptible subjects and prejudice the cardiac function of people with coronary heart disease. It may also increase the chances of non-smokers getting leukaemia and a wide variety of cancers.

Despite growing awareness about the health hazards of smoking through various publicity media, statutory warning on cigarette packets, health education campaingns and efforts of voluntary organizations, people particularly young person, still get lured towards lady Nicotine. Today, in most European countries, more than 50 percent of males and over 30 percent of females are smokers. In Asian countries, the rate of smoking varies from 40 percent to 75 percent among males. World tobacco production touched a record high of 5.5 million tonnes in 1976. World wide, consumers spend almost 100 billion dollars annually on 4 trillion cigarettes.

Studies in India

In India, studies carried out by various workers reveal a wide regional variation in the proportion of smokers-from 75 percent of the men in the North and South-East regions to only about 50 percent in the West. About one third of men have been found to get addicted to smoking before reaching the age of 20 years, even though there is a considerable regional variation. In one study by Babu and Chuttani, the prevalence of smoking among students, 12 to 19 years age group was found to be 8.72 percent. Similarly, in a study of medical students in U.P. by Sandell et al almost one third were found to be smokers. There are reasons to believe that during recent years smoking has registered an increase among the student community. Greater attention will have to be paid to curb the menace if we want to attain the goal of 'Health for All by 2000 A.D.'.

Preventive Steps

To encourage communities and nations to undertake greater effort to reduce smoking. World Health Organisation announced 'Smoking or Health - the Choice is Yours' as the theme of WHO Day in 1980. It is high time that effective steps are taken to prevent and control this modern scourge the smoking epidemic. The control measures should include besides health education, legislative and restrictive measures, ban on smoking advertisements, warning on cigarette, bidi and cigar packets, product modification (production of low tar and low nicotine cigarettes), prevention of tobacco cultivation on commercial scale, increase in tobacco taxation, development of public information and public education programmes and finally the smoking cessation programmes at individual , group and community level. International and voluntary health organizations are doing excellent work in this field and need to be encouraged. Besides the WHO, the other international agencies like UNESCO, UNICEF, FAO, ILO, UNDP etc., are also playing their role in this task. Tobacco Research Council in the UK has done valuable research on smoking problem. Similarly, 'The Vigilance of Action on Smoking and

Health (ASH), a voluntary organization has proved extremely useful in the UK. In the USA,'The National Clearing House for Smoking and Health' has been of inestimable value to all countries facing this problem. In India, unfortunately, there is no voluntary organization exclusively devoted to this cause. There exists "The Cigarette (Regulation of Production, Supply and Distribution) Act 1975 and 'The Cigarette Rules 1976 which compel the manufacturers to display the statutory warning namely 'Cigarette Smoking Is Injurious To Helath' on all cartons and packets of cigarettes but a total ban on advertisement on smoking has so far not been imposed.

Inspite of the well-known health hazards of smoking, the habit goes on almost unabated. Like drinking this habit also often starts as a means for mental relaxation under conditions of stress, for masking shyness, to project a particular social image and under the false belief of its beneficial values. Social sanction and social tolerance are the factors which play a significant role in perpetuating this evil. Once it takes firm roots, it becomes difficult to abandon it as it produces many 'withdrawal symptoms' making the person depressed, morosed, sick and 'out of form'.

Health as such is an individual asset. The basic responsibility of guarding this asset against all possible hazards, lies with the individual himself. No one therefore, need fall in the trap of lady Nicotine, no matter how much alluring it may seem outwardly. Remember, next time when you strike a match box to light your cigarette, you may be igniting your on funeral pyre.

Cigars and pipes are dangerous, too

As few as four cigars or four pipefuls of tobacco give the smoker as much toxic substance as ten cigarettes. Doctors at Minnesota University's School of Public Health, in the USA, advised that even people who have never smoked cigarettes, only a pipe or cigars, should avoid these, too.

Chapter–13

Medico-Social Problems of Today's Youth

Abstract

It is high time now to pay immediate attention to the medico-social problems of youth, analyse their aetiology, magnitude and find a solution so that the youth energy can be properly harnessed and given twist in the right direction towards social progress.

'Flaming youth has become a flaming question. And youth comes to us wanting to know what we may purpose to do about a society that hurts so many of them.'

— Franklin D. Roosevelt

And whatever Roosevelt spoke about youth half a century ago, still holds good today. Today's youth is a confused and a bewildered lot.He has been finding it more and more difficult to adjust and adopt himself to the fast pace of social change that has particularly shaken up the last century or so. Widening of generation gap, conflict of moral values, uncertainty about future career and lack of proper guidance have been the real causes of the youth revolution so noticeable all over the world. It has been rightly said that his reckonable youth force is like a flood which must be controlled and shown proper direction, failing which it is likely to sweep away the gains of social progress so far achieved and leave the society struggling in turbulent water. The signs of this have already started appearing in the form of much of the violence, drug abuse, feeling of frustration and aimlessness among the youth. It is high time now to pay immediate attention to the problems of youth, analyse their aetiology, magnitude and find a solution so that the 'youth energy' can be properly harnessed and given a twist in the right direction towards social progress. Rightly, therefore, the United Nations voiced their concern and drew public attention by declaring 1985 as the 'International Year of the Youth' and the World Health Organization adopted 'Healthy Youth: Our Best Resource' as the theme for the World Health Day in 1985'.

Population Explosion

Any problem connected with youth should be immediately taken note of because of their sheer number alone. It is expected that by the turn of this century, the young population in the age group 15 to 24 years will reach some 1,128 million. In India, this age group accounted for 16.6 per cent of our total population in 1971 which increased to 18.6 per cent in 1981, an increase of about 12 per cent. The population explosion itself has been a major factor lending immensity to the problems of youth. It is felt that by solving this problem of 'population explosion' alone, the country will be able to mitigate most of their problems.

Education Policy

Correct educational policy in respect of youth is another major area of our concern. The present system of education has miserably failed to meet the psycho-social requirements of the youth in toto. Until now it has only been providing a passport to their future employment. With growting unemployment, the system has lost this utility and the youth their faith in the education being provided to them. It is desirable that the education should instill in them a sense of responsibility towards themselves, their families and the society at large. It should also give them a sense of belonging, help them make self supporting and a disciplined lot. The National Educational Policy should not overlook the specific needs of the youth.

One of the major causes of frustration among youth has been a growing uncertainty about employment opportunities. There is a felt need to have a comprehensive plan to rehabilitate all unemployed youth and to give priorities to those activities under Five Year Plans which will create maximum employment opportunities. The rush for service which is the ambition of many youths should be stopped and encouragement provided to settle them in business, agriculture, handicrafts and small scale industries either on individual or cooperative basis. For this, necessary guidance, training and financial help should be made available to them.

Health Problems

Youths have fallen victim of certain health problems, multifactorial in origin, with a variety of psycho-social contributory factors. Most of these problems develop during adolscence which is a very crucial transitional phase from childhood to adulthood. This period is fraught with danger to mental health and may result in 'juvenile delinquency'. A juvenile delinquent is one who has deviated from accepted normal behaviour in interpersonal relations and social life and may be labelled as incorrigible, indisciplined, disobedient, immoral or anti-social. A change in socio-cultural pattern resulting into broken homes, unhappy home atmosphere and lack of healthy recreational facilities has been the basic reason for rise in juvenile deliquency in India as elsewhere during the last few decades. The highest incidence is encountered in children aged 15 years and above and the incidence is four to five times more common among boys than among girls.

Sexually Transmitted Diseases

During recent times a world wide concern has been voiced about the growing incidence of Sexually Transmitted Diseases (STD) among teenagers. Surveys carried out by various workers in our country have revealed a high proportional case rate in respect of youth. The Central Health Education Bureau (CHEB), in their pilot study in Government hospitals in Delhi in 1981 found that an overwhelming majority of victims were youths. Similarly another survey carried out in Lucknow reported that 60 per cent of the patients surveyed were students. Most of the patients admitted that they had their first sexual exposure around 18 years of age. Various surveys also reveal that premarital sex is increasingly becoming an accepted way of behaviour. The prostitutes still happen to be the main source of infection in our country although the 'good time girl' has replaced them in many other countries. Lack of proper sex education, inadequate parental supervision, broken homes, lack of healthy recreation, easy availability of sex thrillers and other pornographic materials, easy availability of contraceptive devices and permissiveness have all contributed towards this growing incidence of STD among youth.

Adolescent Girls

Special attention should be paid to the problems of adolescent girls. In many societies the girls have not been provided with same opportunities as in the case of boys in respect of education, health care, employment etc. They are in no way inferior to boys and their education should not be neglected. In 1975, it was estimated that out of 800 million illiterates in the world, majority (60%) were females. Besides general education, the adolescent girls need to be told about their role as would be mothers and governesses of the household and be prepared for the same. Similarly the adolescent boys will also need to be trained for their future role as fathers and heads of the families. Education on planned parenthood emphasising the evils of population explosion and desirability of small family norm must form an indispensible part of education of adolescents of both the sexes.

Drug Addiction

On the drug front, the picture is getting more dismal. It is no wonder, if today's frustrated and neglected youth, with misguided curiosity, seeks a solace in addiction to drugs which are so easily available. Various surveys carried out among college students in our country reveal that a large proportion of them are addicted to drugs. The proportion was found to be 33 per cent and 37.4 per cent respectively among students of Delhi and Calcutta Universities. In U.S.A., it is estimated that 12-20 million people smoke marijuna and 30 to 50 per cent of all high school students have accepted it as an indispensible part of life. It is feared that by the year 2000 AD when 'Health for All' is to be attained, India will be having nearly 15 million drug addicts. Besides the problem of drug addiction, the youth needs to be protected from the health hazards associated with alcoholism and smoking. Efforts on warfooting are required to impart health education and guide the students, teachers, parents, social workers, etc. on various aspects of preventive measures against drug abuse and their role in implementing these measures. Steps need to be taken to addicts, where required. A newer concept in the form of 'Youth Guidance Clinics' may be given a serious thought on similar lines as 'Child Guidance Clinics' for a comparatively younger lot.

Youth and Accidents

The yough should also be cautioned against accidents. Motor vehicle accidents, drowning and burns happen to be the predominant causes of accidental deaths among 5-24 years age group in U.S.A. In India also accidental deaths are on increase particularly road accidents which account for nearly 33 per cent of all accidental deaths. While extraneous factors responsible for such accidents must be controlled, the children and youth should be taught proper road discipline, traffic rules and made accident conscious.

Lastly, the Government through existing schemes, institutions and also various voluntary organisations should pay special attention to the problems of disadvantaged young people (such as those who are illiterate or could not complete their education; rural youth who finds himself at a disadvantage *vis a vis* his urban counterpart in various competitive fields; slum dwellers; mentally and physically handicapped

youth; adolescent social deviants, etc) and rehabilitate them in instilling in them a ray of hope, by assuring them that they are wanted, by guaranteeing them economic independence and by paying prompt attention to various other factors adversely affecting their physical, mental and social development. Any further neglect of our youth will be suicidal on our part and attainment of 'Health for All by 2000 AD' would be a far fetched dream never to be realised.

Chapter-14

Geriatric Population and their Problems

Introduction

Ageing is an universal phenomenon. "Old age" - these very words bring to our mind images of white hair, drooped shoulders, uncertain gait and a sense of isolation. And yet, old age also means a full active life, a lively spirit and delightful hours spent with grand children. In the orient the elders have traditionally enjoyed privilages and were held in high esteem in the society. They have been revered by one and all and their advice has been sought on various social matters ranging from sowing of the next crop to the decision about a marriage in the family or settling a village feud to prescribing a remedy for a stomach-ache. From position of eminence - depending upon their socio-economic status - those who are well in their eighties, direct many an industrial empire, even in developing countries like India. Today in the age profile of population of many societies, where more than 50 percent are below age of 20 years, elderly population are definitely in a minority (1).

Magnitude of the Problem

With advances in fertility control and improvement in health and social services, life expectancy has gone up. This has resulted in increased population of the elderly as well as their total numbers. We are now entering the age of ageing. By the year 2000 AD; the number of world's aging citizens i.e., persons aged 60 years and above is expected to reach 590 million as compared to 307 million in 1970; most of the growth will be posing problems to health planners and administrators, more so in developing countries (2). In India, elderly people constituted 6.5 percent of total population numbering about 43.2 million population in 1981. It is expected that there will be approximately 80 million elderly population in India by 2000 AD (3). Though problems of old age have not assumed great dimension in India, but they are likely to accelerate due to increased life expectancy, more urbanisation, industrialisation and breaking up of joint family systems.

Elderly people are potentially 'at risk' not just because they are old, but because they are mostly disabled or partly disabled. They are vulnerable to disablement from within the territories of their mind, their bodies or their social and physical environment. Although disability in old age is inevitable, much can be done to minimise it. Aging is pot simply a physical process but a state of mind and today we are witnessing the beginning of a revolutionary changes all over the world in this regard.

Disorders of cardio-vasular system are the most prevalent long term diseases causing disability and incapacity among the elderly. The prevalence of these disorders increased with age. Raudolf in their study of rural aged of 50 years and above observed that 6.1 percent of elderly population were hypertensive. Both systolic and distolic blood pressure showed increasing trend in both the sexes with advancement of age. Ray observed that a little over 26 percent of aged were suffering from one or the other disease of cardio vascular system like atherosolerosis, IHD etc. He confirmed that 1, 7, 2, 5 and 1, 8 percent of the population under survey suffered form Angina pectoris, Myocardial infarction and intermittent claudication respectively. Other common ailments old people found to have suffered from were haomorrhoids and varicose veins.

Disease of nervous system are chronic conditions affecting the physical, mental and social well being in the elderly. Cardio vascular accidents are quite common and more so in developed countries like USA and Scandanavian countries. In his study, Ray observed that 3. 5 percent of the subjects were suffering from disorders of central nervous system (7). Eye diseases among geriatric population assume great significance because of reduction in social contact. Cataract is the most common eye ailement among elderly population. Ray in his study of urban elderly found ocular morbidity in 27 per cent of study subjects. Blindness was prevalent in 1.5 percent of the subjects and other important ocular disorders found in the study were cataract (28%), conjuctivitis (5%), corneal opacity (1.8%) and pterygium (1.5%). Disorders of ear, nose and throat interfere with social interaction with family and other community members and geriatric population is no exception. In a multicentric study of the elderly, sponsored by WHO, prevalence of deafness increased from 20 percent in young population to 70 percent in elderly (6). Disoders of genitourinary system, though more common among elderly are found less frequently in routine surveys, possibly due to lack of facilities for thorough clinical examination. Ray in his survey reported that 2.7 percent of study population had hydrocele and 3 percent suffered from benign hypertrophy of prostrate. Other common diseases found in the survey were urinary tract infection among female population (2.7%) and hernia (0.3%) (8). Disorders of locomotor system leading to falls are quite common in old age and 90 percent of fracture femur specially among females are caused by falls. Osteoporosis is one of the reasons for the fracture. Various workers reported prevalence of osteoarthritis ranging between 10 and 26 percent (9).

Diabetes mellitus and impaired glucose tolerance are common conditions among elderly and more so in obese individuals. Prevalence of diabetes mellitus in Indian studies varied between 1.2 to 14.8 percent (10). Elderly people are subjected to both obesity and undernutrition. Many factors affect intake of nutrients and subsequently nutritional status of the elderly.

Physical Health

The medical problems of old age are far too many and are characterised by multiplicity and chronicity. Reduced mobility due to osteoarthritis, gout etc coupled with failing eyesight and hearing transforms minor tasks into major ones and also reduce the social contacts. Even trivial accidents can become cause for much morbidity and sufferings. The elderly people are also subjected to inevitable illnesses, due to chronic and degenerative diseases like Diabetes, Arthritis, Hypertension etc.

Although main health problems of the geriatric population do not fundamentally differ from those of other age groups, never-the-less ill health in the elderly are manifested by a variety of physical and mental defects, which are generally of long term nature. Morbidity among elderly should not only be assessed in terms of extent of the pathological process but also in terms of impairment of functions, due to underlying causes. From the individual treatment point of view, accurate diagnosis is essential but from the point of planning of health services for them, the disability is considered more important. Chronic conditions have different implications for different people at different ages in terms of disability and hence the physical health in elderly has to be assessed alongwith the limitations of a activities of daily living (ADL) viz bathing, dressing, going to toilet, continence, feeding etc (4).

Medical Problems.

As mentioned earlier, aging is associated with increasing prevalence of chronic diseases and disabilities and their prevalence increases with age. Common diseases encountered among elderly population are enumerated in succeeding paragraphs.

Diseases of teeth and gum are quite common. Various studies revealed that more than 70 percent of elderly aged 60 years and above were eduntalous and more than 7 percent had suffered from dental caries. About 30 percent had periodentel diseases (5). Rajet found that 4.2 percent of the geriatric population were suffering from diarrhoea and gastroenteritis (4). However, constipation is one of the commonest complaints in elderly. In his series, Raj reported that 2.8 percent elderly population were confirmed cases of peptic ulcers and more than 10.5 percent of his study subjects had either nutritional glossitis, cheilosis or angular stomatitis. In all, 27.8 percent of the elderly were found to be suffering from various diseases of alimentary system (5).

Respiratory disoders are more frequent among elderly population. Chronic bronchitis and broncial asthma being the most common ailment, Niyogin ali (6) in their survey in urban area reported that 16 and 5 percent of men and women were suffering from chronic bronchitis and bronchial asthma respectively. Emotional stress, poor housing, poor dentition, diminished sense of taste and smell and physical discomfort, obesity, though quite common in developed countries, is increasing to a great extent in higher socio-economic groups of developing countries. However, undernutrition affects majority of elderly population in developing countries.

Mental Health

Mental illnesses are of significance because of the disability and hardship they give rise to in the afflicted persons as well to their families and the community. The individual will be dependent for many years to social suppot.

Various workers in India have reported prevalence of different mental diseases amongst elderly ranging from 60 to 190/1000 (11). Common psychiatric aliments encountered among geriatric population are senile dementia, affective disorders, anxiety state and schizophrenia. The prevalence increased as age advanced and was found to be more common among illiterates. There are two major components for causation of mental illnesses in elderly-ie. biological and social factors. Former group includes pathological conditions mainly the degenerative process of aging. The factors contribute to ailments such as dementia and psychiatric sequelae of failing eye sight and hearing and slow locomotion. Social factors include bereavment, social isolation, feeling of loneliness, inability to adapt and cope with rapidly changing environmental circumstances and the inadequacy of society's attitude towards elderly members (11).

Social Aspects

In the past, the social system in India provided the care and security that aged people required. Old age was traditionally regarded as a repository of knowledge, virtues and wisdom. Our culture demands that elders should be respected, In fact, the order of precedence in India was mother, father, teacher and God. Since time immemorial, traditional families cling last to the belief that since it is the duty of the parents to look after the dependent parents and by this one pays one's debt to the parents and also paves one's way to salvation. Besides, religious beliefs and traditions being strong in Indian societies, respect for the aged was something that was considered sacred.

Our predominently rural agrarian society is slowly giving way to urbanisation, industrialisation and individualism. Joint family system, where in the young and the old, the employed and the unemployed lived in idyllic harmony, has caved in and the bonds of love and respect for each other is fast disappearing. This problem is further aggravated due to migration of rural youth to neighbouring urban areas in quest of better job and easy life, which has led to loss of family support in rural areas. In urban areas, the economic inadequacies of the nuclear family system is depriving it of the obligation of providing social security to its members specially to the aged, Retirement from work, demise of the spouse, reduced or loss of income, considerable increase in leisure time and the generation gap add to the stressful situation and also pose new problems for adjustment in old age.

Aging is an established social problem in developed countries, where family ties and sentimental attachment have been given a burial. Due to various changes in the social system, this is emerging as an important problem in India as well.

Economic independence has a profound effect on the physical and social health. Adequacy of income results in better nutrition and better utilisation of health care resources. Sudden loss of income which is more common among elderly population in western countries may lead to various psychiatric problems and nervous breakdowns.

Socially, elders are still well integrated. Joint family system serves as an insurance for elders and reduces the prevalance of mental illnesses among them. Small family norm, urbanisation, industrialisation, stress on individualism and glamourising of youth may lead to certain loss of status of the aged in the communities in years to come. Most elderly in India, though they have physical disability are still active participants in spiritual activities. Society should remember that "Youth gives you vision, old knowledge and wisdom".

Chapter–15

Anaemia in Pregnancy

Abstract

Anaemia in pregnancy is preventable to a great extent with supplementation of iron and folic acid. But it is because of certain medical and socio-economic factors that the situation of this group remains so precarious. These factors include multiple pregnancies, worm infestations, poverty, ignorance, illiteracy, poor health education, malnutrition and poor living conditions. Anaemia during pregnancy is, therefore, usually multifactorial in its genesis.

Introduction

Every society regards mothers as an embodiment of love and affection. A Jewish proverb says:

'God could not be everywhere and therefore, He made Mothers.'

-- Anon

In spite of all the reverence shown towards mothers, it is a pity that in today's world, they remain a neglected lot as far as their health and nutrition are concerned. This is evident from the fact that the maternal mortality claimed nearly 5,00,000 lives in the world during 1983. The major brunt was borne by the developing countries which accounted for nearly 4,94,000 deaths. A further analysis of various causes of high morbidity and mortality among mothers reveals that anaemia (particularly nutritional anaemia) is one of the chief culprits responsible for it. Pregnant women are highly vulnerable to this malady. A recent estimate reveals that anaemia afflicted nearly 63.6 million pregnant women in the developing countries. Even in industrialized countries, it did not spare nearly 2.5 million pregnant women. In Asia alone, up to 40 per cent pregnant women have been reported to be anaemic.

Situation in India

Various surveys carried out in our own country shows that nearly 50 to 60 per cent of women suffer from anaemia during their last trimester of pregnancy mainly due to iron and folic acid deficiency. It has been associated with high incidence of premature births, abortions, still-births, low birth weight babies, increased neonatal deaths, puerperal sepsis and thrombo-embolic phenomena in the mother. Pregnant women who are anaemic often suffer from postpartum haemorrage and deliver babies who are also anaemic at birth. Such anaemic mothers also generally take a longer time to recover from infections. Anaemia was found to be the principal cause responsible for 35 per cent of the total maternal deaths. A longitudinal survey carried out at the Medical College Hospital, Nagpur, between 1955 and 1964 revealed that 20 to 40 per cent of maternal deaths were attributable to anaemia. Anaemia is, thus, one of the leading causes of maternal mortality and pregnancy wastage in India. Mudaliar from Madras was one of the earliest workers to draw attention to the high maternal mortality due to anaemia.

Women in reproductive age form a vulnerable group with regard to anaemia. They are susceptible mainly because of their increased nutritional requirements. Ante-natal mothers are regarded as 'high risk' cases as their haemoglobin level is found to be 50 per cent and below than normal expected value. 'Risk approach' is being adopted in providing special, improved maternal and child care to such cases.

Although anaemia in pregnancy is preventable to a great extent with supplementation of iron and folic acid, it is because of certain medical and socio-economic factors that the situation of this group remains so precarious. These factors include multiple pregnancies, worm infestations, poverty, ignorance, illiteracy, poor health education, malnutrition and poor living conditions. Anaemia during pregnancy is, therefore, usually multifactorial in its genesis.

Signs and Symptoms

Anaemia of mild or moderate severity is often missed during pregnancy unless the woman has been attending an antenatal clinic. It's common symptoms include—easy fatiguability and lassitude, breathlessness on exertion, palpitation, dizziness, giddiness, tingling and 'pins and needles' in fingers and toes (paraesthesia), tachycardia, general weakness, in severe cases pain in chest due to exertion (angina pectoris) and an overall decline in the working efficiency of the affected individual. It also adversely affects the immune mechanism of the body and thus increases the susceptibility to infection. The common clinical signs include pallor of the skin, mucous membranes and nails. In severe cases there may be pitting of the nails (koilonychia), oedema of the ankles and crepitations at the bases of the lungs. The diagnosis of anaemia and its type is confirmed by haemoglobin estimation and examination of blood films and bone marrow.

Causes and Treatment

The predominant type of anaemia most commonly encountered during pregnancy is due to iron deficiency which is mainly due to deficient intake of iron in relation to the increased demands of the growing foetus. The other causes may be its poor absorption and assimilation and increased blood losses due to chronic bleeding from some underlying cause. Next to iron, the folic acid deficiency can also cause anaemia. However, in majority of the cases, these two deficiencies are found to be co-existing. The third type of anaemia which is duc to vitamin B_{12} deficiency (megaloblastic or pernicious anaemia) is not so common during pregnancy. The treatment depends upon the nature of nutritional deficiency and its cause such as administration of iron (as ferrous sulphate) and folic acid orally. In severe cases parental iron therapy and even blood transfusion may be required.

Prevention

The curative measures can be better avoided if mothers are prescribed iron and folic acid tablets (each containing 60 mg of elemental iron and 500 mcg of the folic acid) prophylactically as a part of their ante-natal and post-natal care. In routine ante-natal examinations during various contacts, mothers are specially examined for anaemia by carrying out their haemoglobin estimation.

Therapy and prophylaxis with iron and folic acid should always be supplemented with proper advice on diet which should include rich sources of iron. Foods of animal sources providing readily available iron include liver, meat, fish and eggs. Food of plant sources providing iron include cereals, pulses and vegetables particularly the green leafy vegetables. Besides these, iron is also obtained from jaggery, nuts, oilseeds and dried fruits such as raisin, apricots and dates. Milk is however low in its iron content. The suggested dietary intake of iron for Indian women during pregnancy is 40 mg per day and during lactation 32 mg per day. However, daily supplements of 60 mg of iron and 500 mcg of folic acid have been recommended during the second and third trimesters of pregnancy and during lactation. Under MCH Programme, a tablet containing 180 mg ferrous sulphate and 0.5 mg folic acid are administered to pregnant and nursing mothers twice daily after meals until their haemoglobin level is found to be 10-12 g.

Although anaemia happens to be the most important non-obsteric cause of maternal morbidity and mortality in our country, the problem is not insurmountable. Its multifactorial genesis, however, calls for a concerted, intersectoral approach. Besides nutritional supplementation in the form of iron and folic acid tablets, health education of mothers on diet during pregnancy and lactation, regular ante- and post-natal check-ups also need to be emphasised. Prophylactic treatment with iron and folic acid is provided under MCH Programme for nutritional anaemia in women and it was proposed to cover 80 million mothers during the Seventh five year plan period 1985 to 1990.

Mothers should be encouraged to visit MCH clinics conducted by hospitals, Family Welfare Centres, Primary Health Centres and their sub-centres for timely detection and treatment of anaemia and its prophylaxis. There is no doubt that these concerted efforts will definitely help in drastically reducing the maternal mortality in our country which is already too high, *i.e.* 5-10 per 100 live-births as compared to 0.5 per 1000 live births in most of the developed countries. Lastly, we should not forget that it is the mothers only who finally determine the destiny of a nation and of mankind

'For the hand that rocks the cradle
Is the hand that rules the world'.

-- W.S. Ross

Facts for the Safe Motherhood

- Some 500000 women die each year from causes related to pregnancy or childbirth, 99.9% of them in developing countries.
- In many parts of Africa, one woman in 14 dies from the complications of pregnancy or childbirth. The figure is one in 18 in southern Asia. But only one in 4,000 or even one in 10,000 in the industrialized countries. Almost all these deaths are preventable with attainable resources and skills.
- The five leading causes of maternal mortality are haemorrage, abortion, toxaemia (hypertension associated with pregnancy), obstructed labour and infections.
- Four major improvements are needed to enable women to experience motherhood in safety:

  Social equity for women
  Maternity care for all
  Essential obstetrics for those at risk
  Family planning for all couples.
- In 1987 WHO, the World Bank and UNFPA launched an initiative for safe motherhood that also enjoys the

support of UNICEF and UNDP. This initiative is aimed at reducing maternal mortality and morbidity through several complementary activities: advocacy and information dissemination, technical support to countries, epidemiological and operational research and training.

Facts for Breast-Feeding

- Breast milk protects the infant against infection and is the best and cheapest food. Breast-feeding also helps in spacing births.
- Most infants require no other food or liquid than breast milk during the first four to six months of life.
- When the child is four to six months old, breast-feeding needs to be supplemented by cup and spoon-feeding with nourishing and calorie-rich foods from the family meal.
- It is essential to keep up the tradition of breast-feeding where it exists and to revive it where it is dying out. There are curently encouraging trends in this direction.
- In many parts of Africa and Asia, particularly in rural areas, almost all children are breast-fed. In western Europe the percentage of breast-fed children had fallen to only 30% in 1970, but has since risen nd in certain countries is up to 90%.

Chapter-16

Cancer Cervix : The Scourge of Womankind

Abstract

Cancer cervix, by virtue of its accessibility, is one of the most easily diagnosed cancer, if detected in its early stage before metastasis has ocurred. At an early stage, it is the most vulnerable but radical treatment ends with a high cure rate. The unfortunate delay on the part of the patient to report for investigation and delay on the part of medical attendant in diagnosing it often culminates in a poor prognosis.

Introduction

The word 'cancer' or 'carcinoma' literally means a crab. Like a crab, the disease cancer will not easily dislodge itself from its firm grip on the tissues involved. Moreover, unlike a crab, the cancer cells are notorious to spread and evade the distant parts of the body; this process is known as metastasis which makes it invincible to cure. This disease of great antiquity mentioned in 'Papyrus Ebers', the oldest medical literature (1500 BC) afflicts both sexes. However, due to anatomical variations certain cancers are bound to be sex specific. Cancer uterine cervix (commonly referred to as cancer cervix) occupies a unique place among all female malignancies and has been described as the biggest curse of the womankind. Let us see why?

According to a report published by WHO in 1987, an estimated 4,60,000 new cases of cancer cervix occur in the world every hour. The hospital statistics during the period 1968-77 from Indian subcontinental countries of Burma. Nepal and Sri Lanka show that cancer cervix topped the list among the neoplasms and occupied a second place in India and Bangladesh with its percentage varying from 24.4 to 45.3 per cent.

Risk Factos in Cancer Cervix

Studies carried out in India and abroad suggest several risk factors which make a woman more vulnerable to this malady. These risk factors include-poor genital hygience, early marriage, early coitus, multiple sexual contacts and repeated child births. The other contributory risk factors include low socio-economic status, illiteracy, lack of health, poor education/awareness on this subject, increasing span of life and lack of diagnostic and treatment facilities. A large number of our female population is found vulnerable to cancer cervix due to these risk factors. The disease has, therefore, rightly been regarded as multi-factorial in its origin.

Early detection and treatement

Cancer cervix, by virtue of its accessibility, is one of the most easily diagnosed cancer if detected in its early stage before metastasis (distant spread) has occurred. At an early stage it is most vulnerable to radical treatment and also with a high cure rate. Despite this and the fact that the presenting symptoms are relatively dramatic and risk factors so well known, the unfortunate delay on the part of the patient to report for investigation and delay on the part of medical attendant in diagnosing it often culminates in a poor diagnosis. Tremendous progress has been made in the field of early diagnosis of cancer cervix since the invention of vaginal speculum by Marion Sims in 1908. For example, Papanicolaou and Traut's classic discovery of 'Diagnosis of uterine cancer by vaginal smear' in 1943 made it feasible to detect cancer cervix even in its presymptomatic phase. The other discoveries prior to it include : (i) the screening technique of examining the intact cervix under binocular magnification by Hans Hinselman in Germany in 1924 which led to the invention of colposcope in 1925-an essential diagnostic tool, complimentary to cytology in early diagnosis of cancer cervix and (ii) methods for detecting cervical cancer by exfoliative cytology independently by Babes in Vienna and Papanicolaou in United States in 1928. With these advances, today it is possible to detect 70 per cent or more of the cervical diseases including cancer in situ or as early invasive lesion under various screening programmes.

On the treatment side also, tremendous progress has been made. According to Greenwood, a British epidemiologist and statistician, the survival rate in untreated cases of cancer cervix was five years. However, on prompt detection before metastasis has occurred, a woman can now expect to live her normal life span following the radical cure. Besides radical hysterectomy, first performed by Clark in 1885 and popularized by Vertheim in 1905, radium therapy was also been issued used since 1903 for its treatment with reports of long term cure.

Prevention and Control

In the light of aforesaid, the true strategy to be adopted for the prevention and control of Cervical cancer must pay particular attention to the following aspects:-

1. Health education to promote awareness among women, particularly those 'at risk' so that they remain under regular periodic surveillance and report promptly on suspicion of a symptom suggestive of cancer cervix such as bleeding per vaginum which is irregular or abnormal (intermenstrual, postcoital, post menopausal or excessive). vaginal discharge (blood stained or otherwise), pain or incontinence of urine. More effective and greater utilisation of various mass media such as newspapers, magazines, radio and TV, etc., should be made to achieve this aim. Health education must lay emphasis on personal hygienes of the genitalia.

2. Reorientation of medical professionals by inculcating high degree of suspicion of cervical cancer in a woman reporting with symptoms suggestive of it and necessity for thorough clinical examination and investigations to rule out/confirm its possibility.
3. Provision of adequate facilities for early diagnosis through health care delivery system upto the most peripheral level and adequate treatment facilities in referral hospitals.
4. Improvement in cervical cancer registration system which may help as a useful tool for future epidemiological studies and in knowing the trend of the disease.

Lastly, it is needless to stress that the ultimate goal of controlling this scourge of womankind by early detection and prompt radical treatment can only be achieved through a multipronged attack on this disease of multi factorial etiology by controlling/eliminating the well known 'risk factors', adoption of family planning practices and overall improvement in the socio-economic status of the woman.

Chapter—17

Diarrhoeal Diseases among Children: Their Present Status and Our Concern

More than 3 decades ago on 20th November 1959 the United Nations unanimously adopted the Declaration of the rights of the child and affirmed that "all children will be entitled to special protection, opportunities and facilities to enable them to develop in a normal and healthy manner with freedom and dignity"[1]. This affirmation still remains a promise to be fulfilled when assessed against a single, preventable and major cause of high morbidity and mortality among them i.e., the diarrhoeal diseases.

According to UNICEF, almost 2/3rds of the 14 million child deaths each year (8.51 million deaths for 60%) are attributable to just 4 major causes — diarrhoeal diseases, respiratory infections, measles and neonatal tetanus. Out of these, the diarrhoeal diseases alone account for 4 million deaths or 28% of total mortality annually among them[2].

Although reliable data on the incidence of diarrhoeal diseases in our country are not available, since unlike cholera, all those diseases are not notifiable. However, various studies carried out in various parts of our country suggest that on an average, children below 5 years of age suffer from 2 episodes among children of all age groups may be around 500 million per year. Approximately 10% of these episodes lead to dehydration which if untreated become life threatening in 1-2% of cases[3].

Diarrhoeal diseases affect children of all age groups although children below 2 years of age (infants and toddlers) are more susceptible[3, 4]. Breast-fed infants show some amount of resistance to various infections in general and diarrhoea in particular due to inherent immunological properties of human milk[5]. Artificially-fed infants are 3 times more prone to contact diarrhoeal infections.

The various cycle between malnutrition and diarrhoea is already well known. Malnutrition's main victims are children under the age of 15 years who are worst hit. At least 0.5-1 million children die every year in our country due to diarrhoea out of which 25% mortality occurs in children below 5 years of age[6].

Health surveys conducted in rural India show the incidence rate for diarrhoea as 33% and various admission rates as 3.30% to 28.37% in various States for all age groups[7]. Most of these cases may be the source of infection to the children particularly in cases of infective type of diarrhoea. Over 25 different pathogens have been found responsible for causing diarrhoeal diseases[3]. The mode of transmission of these agents is usually through contaminated food, water and milk. Illiteracy/low levels of education and absence of health awareness and health education among mothers and other family members are also some important underlying contributory factors, which call for an urgent social action.

Since, nearly 60% of diarrhoeal deaths among children are consequent to resultant dehydration, the advent of oral rehydration therapy (ORT) has been regarded as the most important single achievement in reducing the mortality[2]. The life of about 50% dehydrated, moribund children can be saved by timely administration of oral rehydration salts (ORS) or their home made substitutes which can also be used as supplements to ORS. These home available fluids (HAF) include sugar-salt solution, butter milk, rice water, *dal* soup, green coconut water, diluted milk and weak tea. ORS packets are available free through government health facilities and on payment from the drug stores[2, 8].

The National Diarrhoeal Disease Control Programme (NDDCP) launched during 1981 in our country emphasised upon reducing the diarrhoea associated childhood mortality to half (50% reduction) by 1990. The strategy adopted to achieve this aim included a 3-tier programme i.e., home management of diarrhoea with HAF for prevention of dehydration, rehydration of mild and moderately dehydrated children with ORS by peripheral health workers and treatment of severe dehydration at health workers and treatment of severe dehydration at health centre/hospital with ORS/IV fluids by the doctor. The 3-tier strategy had to be adopted due to inadequate production of ORS packets initially. Now the Government of India has advocated a switch over to 2-tier system in which the ORS packets procured from WHO/UNICEF can be used even in the prevention of dehydration during its home management[6].

In the light of aforesaid, the present grim picture of diarrhoeal diseases among our children (constituting nearly 40% of our population under 14 years of age) calls for an urgent concerted community/government efforts[9]. In this effort, every doctor has to play a dual role of a treating physician as well as that of a teacher to the community. He/she need not be reminded that the term "doctor" by derivation itself means to teach[5]. As a teacher he/she must impart health education to his/her clients/community on all aspects of prevention against diarrhoeal diseases with special emphasis on ORS. While as a physician, a doctor must keep himself/herself fully conversant with the principles of treatment which have been rationalised including essential steps as follows[4]: (1) Rapidly correct shock and restore hydration. (2) Correct acidosis and potassium loss. (3) Maintain hydration until diarrhoea stops. (4) Reduce further diarrhoea e.g., cholera through appropriate antibiotics. (5) Maintain nutrition.

In the past, training programme for doctors were organised at the district level and orientation courses arranged in collaboration with the Indian Medical Association[10]. It is highly desirable to give further these activities to make the doctors at all levels play an effective role in the success of National Diarrhoeal Diseases Control Programme (NDDCP).

References

1. Central Health Education Burau — The rights of the child. *Swasth Hind* 1978; XXII: 274-84.

2. UNICEF — The State of the World's Children 1990: A Summary, New Delhi: UNICER, 1990: 2, 9.

3. ICMR — National Diarrhoeal Diseases Control Programme, India: Management of Acute Diarrhoea, Calcutta: National Institute of Cholera and Enteric Diseases, 1984: 1.

4. Mahalanobis D — Treatment of Acute Diarrhoeal Diseases in Children. *Indian J Prev. Soc. Med.* 1977; 8: 38-42.

5. Park J.E., Park K., eds. — Textbook of Preventive and Social Medicine. 11th ed. Jabalpur: Banarasidas Bhanot, 1986: 202, 44.

6. Sarkar K, Sircar B.K., Roy S., Deb B.C., Biswas A.B., Biswas R. — Global review on ORT programme with special reference to Indian scence. *Indian J Public Health* 1990: 48, 50.

7. Krishan N.R., Anand A.C., — Acute diarrhoea : A Rational Approach to Diagnosis and Management. *Med. J. Armed Forces India* 1986; 1: 13-9.

8. Central Health Education Bureau — National Health Programmes, *Swastha Hind* 1990; XXXIV: 200.

9. Rama Rao B.R., — The Health of Schol Child. In : Health Action (special issue on mother and child care). Secunderabad : Health Accessories for All (HAFA), 1989: 131.

10. Kapil U — Childhood Diarrhoea : The Deadly Killer, *Swastha Hind,* 1987; XXXI: 94-5.

Chapter–18

Psychosocial Aspects of Hearing Loss

Abstract

Hearing loss, the most desperate of human calamities, places the victim at a great disadvantage. If the victim is young, it may interfere with development of other specialised functions like speech and mental development; and in old age it interferes with social intercourse and deprives one of the companionship which is so vital at this stage.

Introduction

The problem of hearing loss is more than a medical problem with several socio-economic repercussions. Research in normal healthy subjects has revealed that sensory deprivation of any particular modality precipitates catstrophic reactions of the entire organism. The resultant defence reactions are so extensive that virtually every activity of the individual is adversely affected. Sensory deprivation does not limit its effect to the specific modality that has been affected but manifests itself physiologically, psychologically and ultimately sociologically (1).

The social and emotional handicap of deafness needs a great deal of investigation. The incidence of deaf patients in mental hospitals has been noted to be high and breakdown of communication between the deaf person and his environment should be investigated as a factor in mental illness (2). The psychological strain of deafness with its attendants's inability to communicate often results in a withdrawal from society and may lead to paranoid thinking and behaviour (3).

Hearing Loss – a misfortune

Ludwig Van Beethoven is one of history's most outstanding examples of what hearing loss can do to the human spirit. At the age of 28 having already composed over 50 major pieces of music, he began to slowly loose his hearing. In one of his letters he wrote, ".......... how could I declare the weakness of a sense which in me ought to be more acute than in others, a sense which formerly I possessed in highest perfection. My misfortune pains me doubly in that I am certain to be misunderstood. For me there can be no recreation in the society of my fellow creatures, no refined conversation, no interchange of thoughts. Almost alone and only mixing in society when absolutely necessary, I am compelled to live as in exile. If I approach near to people, a feeling of anxiety comes over me lest my condition should be noticed. How humiliating was it when someone standing close to me heard a distant flute, and I heard nothing, or a shepherd singing and again I heard nothing. Such incidents almost drove me to despair; at times I was on the point of putting an end to me life for deprived hearing". His loss was very gradual and progressive. By the age of 48, Beethoven lost his hearing completely. Even so, he continued to write music although he could not hear it performed.

Another notable example is of Helen Keller who was both deaf and blind. To quote her, "I am just as deaf as I am blind". The problems of deafness are deeper and more complex, if not more important than those of blindness. Deafness is a much worse misfortune. For it means the loss of the most vital stimulus, the sound of the voice that brings language, sets thoughts astir, and keeps us in the intellectual company of the man"

Mental and social isolation

Deafness or blindness separates the person from his fellowmen. Behaviour depends on the interaction between the person and the environment. A sensory defect intercepts the passage of certain stimuli and thus interferes with the interaction between the individual and his environment. For the deaf, sound waves (the chief mode of communication) are unable to get through, hence the person is unable to understand other people adequately: and since we learn to talk by imitation, the deaf also have difficulty in learning to speak and, therefore, are unable to express themselves adequately. In the case of the blind, light rays (the chief guide in personal motility and the source of much pleasure) are unable to penetrate and hence the individual is seen apart from his fellowmen by his lack of freedom of movement and his inability to share the pleasure of seeing. Either deafness or blindness is such a strong barrier that the person can neither break through it nor go over it and only under certain conditions can he go around it by long circumnavigation (use of other senses after specialised training). Thus the handicapped individual lives behind a barrier which interferes with the complete interaction between himself and his objective environment. His activities are curtailed and his interests diverted and hence his behaviour differs from that of his fellowmen, because of the isolation from the environment caused by the handicap. The deaf suffers from mental and social isolation and the blind primarily from physical isolation. The above discussion supports the idea that the deaf are more isolated than the blind who are in turn more isolated than the normal. This view is also in conformity with the personal experience of Helen Keller noted above which made her endorse that the problems of deafness are deeper and more complex than that of blindness.

To elucidate this point further it must be stated that in the adult even after the normal development of language, words must still be heard and understood if ideas are to be accurately expressed. Words play an enormous part in our lives. They have the power to mould our thinking. Social relationships are very often seriously affected as a result of impaired communication. The older we get the greater is the social impact of hearing loss on our lives.

Psycho-educational evaluation

An extensive psycho-educational evaluation was administered to 40 children with hearing impairment to investigate the effects of degree of hearing impairment on intellectual, social, academic and language behaviour. Although children varied greatly in performance, hearing loss of any degree appeared to affect psycho-educational development adversely leading to the conclusion that even minimal hearing loss places children at risk for language and hearing problems.

To conclude, it may be stated that hearing loss is a handicap which has been rightly called "the most desperate of human calamities" by Samuel Johnson. It places the victim at a great disadvantage. If young, it may interfere with development of other specialised functions like speech and mental development; if in the old age, it interferes with social intercourse and deprives one of the companionship which is so vital at this stage. Psycho-social research pertaining to social adjustment and personality development of the deaf has not infrequently produced conflicting or inconsistent findings. Part of this can be due to methodological deficiencies. In the midst of such grey areas occasional insights into the "silent world" offered by recordings, the victims themselves as in the case of Beethoven and Helen Keller can help us understand the complex problems of the deaf considerably, though generalization can still be hazardous.

Chapter-19

Population Explosion : A Self Inflicted Catastrophe

The world's population was around 250 million only about 200 years ago. It became 798 million in 1800 AD; 1650 million in 1900 AD; 2526 million in 1950 and crossed 5000 million mark on 11 July 1987. Now 11th July every year is observed as World Population Day. The ever increasing rate of population growth has now reached a stage where it is more appropriate to call it as population explosion. According to Dr. U Ko Ko, former Regional Director of WHO SEA Region "Never before in the history of the human race has mankind faced the kind of ecological uncontrolled urbanization and industrialization which have brought in their wake widespread pollution of air, water and land as well as deforestation, desertification, accidents involving chemicals, and the danger of extinction of some plant and animal species. In the name of progress, man seems to have thrown caution to the winds. All that matters is the perceived benefit in the short term".

No doubt, population explosion is a self-created catastrophe which the mankind has brought upon itself. It has been aptly described as a suicidal act by many population experts since its consequences are going to be disastrous in the near future. It has been regarded as the basic cause for consistently wiping out at an increasing pace the existing global resources considered essential for the very survival of the mankind besides many other living species. Since it has been found mainly responsible for creating the gross ecological imbalance unfavourable for their growth and development, let us examine in brief why population explosion is being incriminated as a suicidal act.

Food

Food is very essential for growth and development of every human being right from its birth till he survives. Today, the picture on the food front is very grim. There is neither enough land nor more advanced technology to feed an additional 92 million mouths which get added to world population every year. In 1987, world reserves of grain were sufficient for 101 days. In 1989, there was enough grain stored for 54 days only. The gradual loss of topsoil is important in this context. For every inch of topsoil lost, yield falls by 6% resulting into a total loss of 24 billion tonnes each year. Besides this, nearly one million acres of land is also lost each year as houses are being built. Moreover an individual should have adequate money to purchase food to meet his own requirement and that of his family members. Here again the picture is very gloomy. According to the World Bank estimates about 800 million people in the world are "absolutely poor" — the equivalent of the total populations of the erstwhile USSR, the USA and the whole of Western Europe. Malnutrition, the eternal sign of poverty still remains one of the most persistent of the health problems of the urban poor. According to WHO, the energy and protein intakes of some 145 million children under 5 years of age are still insufficient. Malnourishment predisposes children to infections and diarrhoeal diseases. It is hard to grasp that nearly five million children die from diarrhoeal diseases every year in the third world alone.

Shelter

Besides food (a balanced diet), every individual needs a proper shelter. According to WHO (1987), "Although precise statistics are not available, over 100 million people have no shelter at all, while around one billion lack an adequate shelter". According to UN data, in Latin America and Carribean alone there are 40 million children who lack proper shelter and are living on streets.

Majority of the world population still depends on wood for cooking of food and for provision of proper shelter. Forests are the main source for providing this item. The ever increasing demand of wood is causing fast destruction of tropical forests mentioned as "earth's lungs" — at the rate of one hectare in every 2 to 2.5 minutes. During 1989 alone, 28 million acres of tropical forests were destroyed.

Population explosion has also been found the root cause in the genesis of some major problems of environmnental concern such as global warming (green house effect), Ozone layer depletion, acid rains, air and water pollution, improper waste disposal, etc., appropriately described as manmade wounds to our Mother Earth.

All above considerations thus justify the conclusion that the population explosion is nothing but a suicidal act for which mankind itself is to be blamed. If mankind wants to save itself and save the Mother Earth, it has to be act now otherwise it may be too late. The action required calls for an honest and more vigorous implementation of various strategies suggested for population control at global level and at the same time a determined effort to improve upon socio-economic conditions and to prevent the environmental degradation causing ecological imbalance which may be responsible for the loss of nearly one tenth of all species by the turn of the Century and nearly one third by the year 2020 A.D. The World Population Day (11 July) every year is a perpetual reminder that:

"The need of the hour is to launch a revolution,
To curb the population, poverty and pollution".

References

1. "'Population Reports", Series M. Vol XX, No. 2 May 1992.
2. "World Health Statistics", Vol 44, No. 4, 1991.
3. "British Medical Journal", Vol. 4, No. 12, Feb. 1989.
4. "Test Book of Preventive & Social Medicine" by Park JE & Park K, 13th edn. 1991.

Chapter–20

Intestinal Helminthiasis – A Scourge to Humanity

Abstract

Intestinal helminthiasis forms one of the significant public health and clinical problems in our country. A typical clinical manifestations including eosiaophilic pneumonitis, peptic ulcer syndrome, neuro ocular cysticercosis and stunted growth in children are not uncommonly observed. Early recognition and specific antihelminthic therapy together with supportive therapy tend to control the morbidity associated with disease.

Introduction

Despite the high prevalence of intestinal helminthic infestations in our country, it has not received the attention it deserves. Easily spreading bacterial and viral infections always took priority, in view of its life threatening course of illness. The insidious but chronic ill health caused by most of the parasitic infections hence do not cause an epidemiological threat. Inadequate health education, lack of compliance on the part of the population-more so children being the most vulnerable group exposed to infection-to attend to the hygienic measures together with poverty, overcrowding and poor sanitation add problems to the clinicians and opidemiologists in the control of this continuing challenge. The purpose of this communication is to briefly review the problems, confronted in a developing country like ours, with special reference to the common infestations from a clinician's angle.

The common intestinal helminths infesting the country's population include the following:-

(a) Nematodes: Ascaris lumbricoides (round-worms), Ankylostoma duodenale and Necator Americanus (hook-worms), Strongyloid stercoralis, Trichuris trichura and Enterobius vermicularis.

(b) Cetsodes: Taenia solium, Taenia saginata, (Tapeworms)

Magnitude of the Problem

It is estimated that nearly 3000 million people will be victims to human helminthiasis by the year 2000 unless efficient functioning of primary health care as per the WHO strategy is ensured. A review undertaken 32 years after Stoll's paper on 'This wormy world' revealed that ascariasis and hook-worm disease were classed among the 2[illegible] infections causing the highest morbidity rates. Infection with intestinal parasites may remain asymptomatic for long periods or can present with a number of ill asymptomatics for long periods or can present with a number of ill defined gastrointestinal features, at times mimicking peptic ulcer disease, stunted growth, undernutrition and/or pulmonary eosinophilia. Not uncommonly it may present as intestinal obstruction, gangrene of gut volvulus, granulomatous peritonitis and/or obstructive jaundice. Adult worms have been seen in eustachian tube, bile duct, paranasal sinuses and cavity of heart.

Different health surveys conducted in various urban and rural area in India in recent years revealed that the prevalence or enteric parasitosis ranged from 42 to 66 percent. Most of the workers reported that the general prevalence appeared to rise with increase in age, adults showing a high prevalence of 69.6 percent, one third of them having mixed infestations.

In a multicentric armed forces study, the overall prevalence of intestinal helminthiasis has been reported to the 59.19 percent. Various morbidity statistics indicate that the disease states claim about five million lives every year while another fifty million people suffer from the disease. The distribution of infestations in different areas is given in table 1.

Table 1. Prevalence of intestinal parasitic infections in various surveys

Sr. No.	Authors	Place of survey	Year	Population covered	Entamoeba hystolytica (%)	Giardia Lamblia (%)	Ascaris lumbricoides nale (%)	Ankylostoma duodecularis (%)	Enterobius Vermi- (%)	Trichuris trichiura (%)	Tacnia solium	Prevalence rate (%)
1	2	3	4	5	6	7	8	9	10	11	12	13
1.	Kulkarni et al (6)	Seven villages around Nagpur	1978	2353	30.7	18.3	11.6	27.8	-	-	-	-
2.	Srachari Rao (4)	Urban area	1975	1057	22.8	-	34.2	-	-	4	-	56.4
3.	Yunus et al (5)	Rural area in UP (Aligarh)	1978	2938	20.1	-	22.1	-	-	-	-	42.2
4.	Paul et al (15)	Rural area in Arunachal Pradesh	1981	400	13.9	15.9	45.0	0.4	-	45	74.1	
5.	Rao et al (16)	Urban area in Delhi	1970	327	19.6	23.5	0	0	0	0	0	60.3
6.	Rao et al (17)	Rural area in Mahasu Dt. U.P,	1970	Not known		7.4	7.4	33.3	13.5	-	-	- -
7.	Varma (7)	Eight service centres	1982	816	0.37	9.80	18.99	32.84	-	4.19	1.35	59.3

Ascaris Lumbricoides

It has a wider world prevalence in humid tropical countries (20-98% population in various countries). The female worm is extremely prolific; the eggs deposited in soil are resistant to antiseptic, heat and dryness. The infection is acquired by ingesting embryon and eggs. The larval stage, while passing through lung causes features of 'eosinophilic pneumonitis' or Loffler's syndrome; less often it mimicks tropical eosinophilic syndrome which fortunately is short lived, benign and amenable to anthelminthic therapy. It has been found that 20 adult ascaris can consume 2.8 g of carbohydrate daily.

Heavy ascaris infection gives rise to toxaemic features with dehydration and intestinal obstruction (volulus, gangrene or gut intususception) and appendicitis. Haemorrhagic pancreatitis, cholangitis, choleycystitis, perforation of bile duct are rarc complications. In patients with ascariasis with small bowel obstruction, fragmentation of worms mass and massaging of worms onwards into large bowel is preferred to removal of worms by enterostomy. Masses of adult worms may show up a filling defect on barium meal examination. Diagnosis is confirmed by demonstration of the worm or eggs in stool or larvae in the sputum. Periodic mass therapy given three times yearly for a period of three years, using broad spectrum anthelminthics is the most effective method of control (table 2).

Ankyolstoma duodenale and Necator americanus (Hookworms)

The severity of infection is based on average eggs per gram of stools for the community. Paticnts excreting more than 5000 eggs/gm of facces are considered to be having hookworm disease. The infection is caused by gaining entry of filariform larve, through skin, which passes through lung and settle in the upper intestine. The majority of patients presents with lassitude, dyspnoae, abdominal symptoms, loose stool and other features of iron deficiency anemia. Hookworm dermatitis at

Table 2 Anthelminthic drugs : Therapeutic efficacy

Sr. No.	*Drug*		*T. Solium/ sagninata*	*Ascaris*	*Hookworm*	*Entcrobius*	*Trichutis*	*Strongloids*
1.	Piperazine Salts	100 mg/kg	-	+++	+	+++	-	-
2.	Pyrantel Pamoate	10 mg/kg	-	+++	++	+++	-	-
3.	Oxantel Pamoate	10 mg/kg	-	++	++	+++	-	-
4.	Mebandazole	100 mg/b.d. 3d	-	++	++	+++	++	+
5.	Thiabendazole	25 mg/kg	-	++	++	++	+	+++
6.	Levamisole	5 mg/kg	-	+++	+	+	-	-
7	Pyrvinium	5 mg/kg	-	+	-	+++	-	-
8.	Bephenium OH naphthoate	2.5 g	-	-	+++	-	-	-
9.	Niclosamide	0.5 g BDX 2d	++	-	-	-	-	-
10.	Fraziquantel	50 g mg/kg	+++	-	-	-	-	-

the site of entry through the skin and congestive cardiac failure are uncommon features. Some may complain of anginal pain and pulmonary symptoms suggestive of tropical eosinophila. Eosinophilia not uncommonly persists even after deworming, probably due to stimulation of bonemarrow. In addition to anaemia, features of malabsorption leads to loss of protein and other nutrients. Barium meal examination may show thickened duodenal mucosal folds and widened jejunal loops with coarse irregularity, mottling and patchy appearance. Infestation with ankylostoma is more harmful than necator which is increasingly noticed in South India. Good nutrients and haematinics are desired to be given for longer periods even after control of infection. In patients with severe anaemia leading to cardiac failure, one or two units of packed red cells or parenteral iron may be given to enable early recovery and reduce hospitalisation. Replacement oral iron therapy is to be given 2-3 months after correction of the deficiency. Specific therapy is aimed at eradication of infection by 2 or 3 daily doses of bephenium hydroxynaphtoate 5 g (2.5 g) base given with syrupy juice early morning. Bitoscante 100 mg twice for children and thrice for adults at intervals of 12 hours is more beneficial in patients with necator infection. Mabendazole 100 mg. twice daily for 3 days is an alternate drug employed in resistant cases.

Strongyloids Stercoralis (Dwarf tape worm)

The infection is caused by penetration of infective form through skin or by auto-infection through bowel mucosa or perianal skin. When they inhabit upper gut, patient presents with colicky abdominal pain, diarrhoea or features mimicking tropical sprue syndrome, Irritability and deformity of duodenum due to duodenitis may otherwise simulate duodenal ulcer. Erythema at the site of entry and eosinophilic pneumonitis are other features caused by the larvae. Diagnosis is made by the demonstration of rod shaped larvae in the stool and rarely in sputum, urine or bile. Thiabendazole 25 mg/kg twice daily for 3 days and pyrvinuim pamoate 5 mg/kg daily for 5-7 days eradicate the infection in the majority of cases.

Trichuris Trichiura (Whip worm)

The infection, mostly benign in its clinical course, is often associated with ascaris infection and reported prevalent all over our country. In heavy infection, patients present with bloody diarrhoea, loss of weight, anemia and rarely volvulus, prolapse rectum and abdominal distention simulating acute abdomen. Diagnosis is established by demonstration of ova in stool. Mabendazole, which may have to be reported, eradicate the infection.

Cestodes

Taenia solium (pork tapeworm) and Taenia saginata (beef tapeworm) are ribbon shaped worms inhabiting human intestinal tract. Larvae liberated from the ova present in mature proglottids are ingested by man by eating under-cooked food. The larvae (cysticercus cellulosae) penetrate the bowel mucosa and lodge in brain, spinal cord, eyes, muscles, subcutaneous tissues and rarely heart.

The ad--lt worms inhabiting intestine manifest with upper abdominal pain, wieght loss and abdominal discomfort.

Taenia solium and Neurocysticercosis

There are increasing reports of neurocysticercosis the manifestations of which develops 5-20 years after the larval deposition in the brain, spinal cord or meninges. The problem remains mainly of prevention and public health, as radical cure for extensive infestation is difficult. By virtue of its diverse and polymorphous clinical profile, it mimicks neurosyphilis, neurotuberculosis and multiple sclerosis. Clinical syndromes include seizures, meningoenoephalitis, pseudotumour cerebri, syndrome of ICSOL, psychiatric manifestations, compressive reticulo myelopathy, ocular cysticereosis causing occasionally blindness and pseudo hypertrophic myopathy. Diagnosis is suggested by examination of stool, CSF, blood (for eosinophila), EEG, pneumo-encephalogram and CAT scan. CT scan has lately facilitated the clinician in detecting the brain lesion even in the quiescent and hypertensive crisis stages. Therapeutic measures include therapy with niclosamide and/or praziquantel for both tapeworm infestations. For cerebral cysticercosis, fraziquantel 50 mg/kg in 2 divided daily dose is given for 10 days starting one day prior to specific therapy. Antiepileptic drugs and bitemporal decompression will be required in patients with seizures and hydrocephalus respectively. Localised cysts can be removed with relative case.

In conclusion, intestinal helminthiasis is one of the continuing public health problems that causes considerable morbidity and occasionally mortality in a developing country like ours. Association of malnutrition often related to the infestation adds problem to the clinician. Improvement in the socioeconomic status together with health education on the pathogenesis and preventive measures, it is hoped, is likely to show decrease in the prevalence of this preventable disorder.

References

1. Davis A: This wormy world. Health 1984 3, 2-3.
2. Benjamin DC: Ascaris: most popular worm. World Health 1984 : 3, 8-9.
3. Gopinathan VP : Clinical profile of intestinal helminthic infections from eastern parts of India J Com Dis 1989; 12(3), 151-55.
4. Connor EB: Latent and chronic infection imported from South East Asia. JAMA 1978, 239. 1901.
5. Yunus M. Zaheer M. Sinha S : Prevalence of intestinal parasites, J Ind. Med. Assoc. 1971; 69: 241-245.
6. Kulkarni SW; Panickerr PVRC; Gadkari AS; Handa BK: Prevalence and pattern of parasitic infections in rural areas around Nagpur. Ind. J. Med. Res. 1978; 68: 583-591.
7. Varma BD : Prevalence of intestinal helminthic parasites among Indian Army recruits. Med. J. Armed Forces Ind. 1984; 40(4) : 197-199.
8. Park JE; Park K: Text book of Preventive and Social Medicine Ninth Ed., Banarasi Das Bhanot. 1983-189.

9. Gopinathan VP: Tropical pulmonary eosinophilia - A clinical study, Med. J. Australia 1983: 1, 69-72.

10. Patel JC: Ankylostomiasis in India - A review with suggestions for future research. Ind. J. Med. Res 1954; 42, 279-304.

11. Edwards CRW: Diseases due to infection. In Davidson's Principles and Practice of Medicine. 14 ed. ELBS/Churchill Livingstone 1984, p 788-794.

12. Venkataraman S; Vijayan GP: Neurocysticereosis in Progress in Clinical Medicine in India IV series. Arnold Heinemann New Delhi 1981, p 382-406.

13. Phatarphod SA: Meishri YV; Pai-dhunghat AJ; Nihalani KD; Cysticercosis - oral, intracranial and cutaneous. J. Assoc. Phys. Ind, 1982; 30, 185-6.

14. Sreehari Rao Y; Sahai BN: Prevalence of intestinal parasitic infection in urban area. Ind. J. Pub. Health 1975; 19 (3): 101-105.

15. Paul RC; Das NC; John VM; Rao CK: Prevalence of intestinal parasitic infection in rural population of Arunachal Pradesh J. Com. Dis. 1982; 14 (4); 309-312.

16. Rao CK; Krishnaswamy AK; Gupta SR; Biswas H; Raghavan NGS: Prevalence of amoebiasis and intestinai parasitic infection in a selected community. Ind. J. Med. Res. 1971; 58: 1365-1372.

17. Rao CK; Krishnaswamy AK; Biswas H: Prevalence of intestinal parasitics in selected villages of Mahasu District. Ind. J. Med. Res. 1971; 59: 1959-1985.

SECTION V
MISCELLANEOUS

Chapter–21

Medico-Social Study of Paraplegics in Armed Forces

Abstract

A cross sectional study of 81 paraplegics was carried out to determine various medical and psychosocial aspects of the disability. Majority of the cases were results of preventable external injuries which mostly affected the young productive age group. A large number of cases had permanent impairment of mobility, bowel, bladder and sexual functions. Psychological reactions of anxiety and denial were most frequently encountered in initial stages, but gradually declined in successive stages of rehabilitation. Individuals with independent vocations were psychologically and socially well adjusted.

Introduction

Paraplegia due to a severe injury or disease of the spinal cord undoubtedly constitutes one of the most devastating calamities of human life resulting in severe disablement which inevitably disrupts the psychosocial entity of the affected individual.

Paraplegia is not just an acute disorder. After the initial damaging blow, chronic and long term effects on the body without a controlling central nervous system are staggering. Mojority of cases are traumatic in origin and hence are absolutely sudden in onset-like a "bolt from the blue". Many of the victims unfortunately are young, virile, and productive adults who are transformed tragically to hopeless invalids. Most of them have to spend rest of their lives in wheel chair or in bed.

Majority of the paraplegics in Armed Forces are young who got affected due to trauma sustained during duty while serving the nation. Their expectations are naturally high and it becomes the moral responsibility of the society to rehabilitate them rightfully as it's useful members.

In this article, an attempt has been made to determine different underlying causes of paraplegia and ascertain the various medical, psychological and social aspects of the disability in the study population.

Material and Methods

A cross sectional study of paraplegics was carried out in mid 80s for a period of six months at the three centres located at Kirkee viz. Spinal Cord Injury Centre at Military Hospital (MH), Paraplegic Home and Queen Mary's Technical School (QMTS). All the 81 cases available during the period formed the material of the study. In order to compare the various stages of rehabilitation, the study population was divided into three groups as shown in figure 1 namely-

(a) Group I - comprised of all paraplegics in Military Hospital Kirkee, undergoing treatment in acute phase.

(b) Group II - consisted of all paraplegics in MH Kirkee who had completed their initial intensive phase of treatment and were undergoing further rehabilitative management, and

(c) Group III - subjects consisted of all paraplegics who were residents of Paraplegic Home and Queen Mary's Technical School. (QMTS). The study population in this group had completed their medical management and were living in these institutions during the study period.

Data was collected on the basis of a carefully pretested schedule. The purpose of this study was explained and all cases were subjected to detailed clinical history and systematic examination. For assessing psycho-social condition, interview and observatin techniques were adopted.

The schedule consisted of three parts:-

(a) Personal characteristics of the subject including age of onset, literacy, trade, marital status etc.

(b) Medical aspects including level of lesion, underlying etiology, mobility, bowel, bladder, sexual functions etc.

(c) Psycho-social aspects including level of anxiety, depression, optimism, withdrawal, social and vocational adjustments.

Findings and Discussion

Age of onset and underlying pathology

Almost all studies on paraplegia bring out the young age of onset (3, 4). This is more so in cases of traumatic paraplegia highlighting accidents as predominant cause to which young people are specially prone. This was also revealed in the present study where 86.4 percent of all cases were between 21 and 40 years of age. The frequency was highest in the 21 to 25 years age group (32.1%) followed by 26-30 years age group (30.8%). In cases of traumatic paraplegia, 72.2 percent were found to be less than 30 years of age. These findings are shown in Table I.

Table I

Frequencey distribution of paraplegics of traumatic and non-traumatic origin according to the age of onset

Age Group	*Traumatic*		*Non-Traumatic*		*Total*	
	No.	*% Age*	*No.*	*% Age*	*No.*	*% Age*
16-20	5	7.0	-	-	5	6.2
21-35	24	33.3	2	22.2	26	32.1
26-30	23	32.9	2	22.2	25	30.8
31-35	11	15.3	-	-	11	13.6
36-40	6	8.3	2	22.2	8	9.9
41+	3	4.2	3	33.4	6	7.4
Total	72	100.0	9	100.0	81	100.0

Similar observations were made by Sutton (5) and Masalawala (6) with 72 percent of cases under 40 years of age and Bracken (7) reported the figures to be 85.4 and 66.2 percent respectively under 44 years of age. In a survey in India, Nagpur Association for the Rehabilitation of Children and Adults with Orthdopaedic and other Disabilities (NARCAOOD) found 72 percent paraplegics to be in 16-45 years age group (8).

The present study revealed a slightly higher proportion of cases in the younger age groups as the Armed Forces population is limited by service requirements to an age group of about 17 to 50 years. However, these findings are in conformity with a similar study on Armed Forces personnel by Varma and Boparai (9) who reported that 84 percent cases were in 21-40 years age group.

Trade and Educational Level

Most of the paraplegics were personnel employed in various technical trades which deal with or operate various machinery and equipment, like vehicle mechanics, electricians etc. and drivers of mechanical transport (49.4%) followed by 'general duty' category (43.2%). Rest belonged to clerical (2.5%) and other trades (4.9%).

Most of the cases in the study were educated upto middle school and above (76.6%). Masalawala (6) reported 47 percent of his cases to be labourers and 'city workers'. Armed Forces, with their inherent mobility and increasing mechanisation pose a greater risk to drivers and technical categories.

Marital Status

Marital status does not seem to affect the onset of paraplegia. Paraplegia on the other hand seems to affect the marital status although not very significantly as per findings of the study. In the present study, two separations were noted among the married subjects (4.2%) after they became paraplegic. However, in one instance, it was also noted that an unmarried subject got married after the onset of paraplegia (3.13%).

Other studies in developed countries have concluded that separation or divorce were not significantly higher amongst paraplegics than in the general population (4, 5, 7, 10).

Causes of Paraplegia

Trauma was the strikingly predominant cause of paraplegia accounting for 88.9 percent of all cases. This is in conformity with 80 to 90 percent traumatic etiology reported by Michaelis (3). Similarly majority of cases reported by Varma and Boparai (9), Guttman (1) and Watson (11) were due to trauma.

Table II depicts the external causes of injury leading to paraplegia.

Table II

External causes of injury leading to paraplegics of traumatic origin

Causes	*Number of Cases*	*Percentages*
Vehicle accident	31	43.1
Sports injury	11	15.3
Act of violence	6	8.3
Fall	15	20.8
War injury	1	1.4
Others	8	11.1
Total	72	100.0

Motor vehicle accidents were found to be the major causes of external injury accounting for 43.1 percent of the traumatic cases in the present series. This is in conformity with findings of Fine et al (4) who also reported 42 percent cases and Verma & Boparai (9) who found 39.9 percent cases due to motor vehicle accidents. The next frequent cause was 'falls' (20.8%) in which majority of cases were sustained in rural area (mostly from trees) while individuals were on leave. Masalawala (6) had reported that 62 percent of cases were due to falls.

It is evident that majority of the external causes of injury are accidental in nature and mostly preventable. Motor vehicle accidents are the commonest specific situation responsible for such injuries. Falls are important causes in the rural setting.

Medical Aspects

Analysis of mobility status of paraplegics in the study population revealed that cases in Group II who had completed their acute phase in management but were still in hospital undergoing rehabilitation training, were best placed mobility wise. 25.9 percent of them could walk with aid and the rest used wheel chair. None were bedridden. Patients in Group I understandably fared the poorest with 50 percent being bed-ridden. Observation of Group III cases, who had completed their hospital management phase, revealed 97.4 percent to be wheel chair borne and only one patient was using crutches. None were bedridden, Patients in Group III could be compared favourably with the findings of other similar studies (5, 10, 12). These series reported 38 to 75 percent wheel chair borne cases; 17 to 48 percent walking with or without aids and 7 to 32 percent bedridden.

Absence of bedridden cases in Group III in the present series signified excellent aftercare services. The proportion of wheel chair borne patients was high because most paraplegics who could walk, with or without aid preferred to return to their home rather than stay in Paraplegic Home.

Table III

Group-wise distribution of paraplegics as per their degree of mobility

Mobility

Group	*Walking with Aid*	*Wheelchair Borne*	*Bedridden*	*Total*
I	2 (12.5%)	6 (37.5%)	8 (50%)	16 (100%)
II	7 (25.9%)	20 (74.1%)	-	27 (100%)
III	1 (2.6%)	37 (97.4%)	-	38 (100%)
Total	10 (12.3%)	63 (77.8%)	8 (9.9%)	81 (100%)

Autonomic Functions

Bladder and bowel control, as well as sexual function was found better in Group II than group III cases because patients with adequate control often were those with incomplete lesions, who also had lesser mobility impairment and preferred to return home after treatment.

The present study also revealed that amongst autonomic dysfunctions, sexual function was the most vulnerable to permanent damage, followed by micturition and lastly defection (Table IV). This is in conformity with findings of Tarabulcy (13.).

Table IV

Functional status of bowel, bladder and sexual function in group III paraplegics

Functional Status	*Percentage of Paraplegics with*		
	Bowel Function	*Bladder Function*	*Sexual Function*
I. Total loss of function/ functional control	18.40	39.50	79.00
II. Partial loss of function/ trained function	79.00	57.90	15.80
III. Normal function	2.60	2.60	5.20
Total	100.00	100.00	100.00

Psycho-social aspects

Anxiety was a predominant psychological factor in the early stages of rehabilitation. With gradual adjustment, level of anxiety decreased progressively from Group I where 50 percent had "extremely high anxiety" followed by Group II (22.2%) and Group III (13.1%). However, no significant change was found in the levels of depression amongst these groups. Thus level of depression persisted in most paraplegics although the anxiety showed reduction with successive stages of rehabilitation. This is in conformity with the findings of Suri (14).

Acceptance to the disability of paraplegia was found to occur gradually in most of the cases. Majority of the subjects were not found to be withdrawn and they co-operated.

Majority of the families of the patients in Group I had not been able to accept the disability (62.5%). However the proportion of such families decreased significantly ($p < 0.05$) with stages of rehabilitation viz. 40.7 percent in Group II and 23.7 percent in Group III.

Table V

Presence of withdrawal, acceptance and optimism amongst different groups of paraplegics

Group	*Number of Cases In Group*	*Number of Cases* *Withdrawal*	*Acceptance*	*Optimistic*
I	16	3 (18.7%)	5 (31.3%)	8 (50%)
II	27	5 (18.5%)	16 (59.3%)	13 (48.2%)
III	38	3 (7.9%)	35 (92.1%)	19 (50%)
Test of	X	0.07	21.39	0.02
signi-	df	1	2	2
ficance	p	0.5	0.001	0.5

Table VI

Factors in Social rehabilitation amongst different groups of paraplegics

Group	*Number of Cases In Group*	*Number of Cases* *Acceptance by Family*	*Social Emba-rrasment*	*Feeling of Loss of Status*
I	16	6 (37.5%)	6 (37.5%)	5 (31.3%)
II	27	16 (59.3%)	13 (48.2%)	17 (63%)
III	38	29 (76.3%)	14 (36.8%)	20 (52.6%)
Test of	X	7.49	0.92	4.05
signi-	df	2	2	2
ficance	p	0.05	0.50	0.10

In contrast the social embarrassment and feeling of loss of status in society experienced by paraplegics showed no significant difference amongst the various groups (Table VI).

All cases belonging to Group III of the present study lived in homes for disabled and not in the community at large. They interacted mostly with other disabled. Hence the effects of social trauma manifested as social embarrassment and loss of status in society persisted.

Vocational Aspects

73.87 percent of Group III paraplegics were found to be employed. This compares favourably with other studies which had reported employment of paraplegics ranging between 30 and 88 percent (15-160).

82.1 percent of the employed paraplegics were working in the sheltered workshop (Table VII).

Table VII

Employment status of Group III paraplegics

	Employed			
	Independent Vocation	*Sheltered Workshop*	*Not Employed*	*Total*
Number	5	23	10	38
Percentage	13.2	60.5	26.3	100.0

Though the sheltered workshop has an invaluable place in rehabilitation - providing motivation, training and entrepreneurship (17). They do not still provide achievement of social integration. Thus those working here still had feelings of social embarrassment and loss of social status. In contrast, all subjects who were pursuing independent vocations outside, were found psychologically and socially well adjusted. They were active participants in the main stream of community life and had thus achieved social integration - the ultimate goal of rehabilitation.

References

1. Guttman L. Spinal Cord injuries-Cord injuries-comprehensive management and research. Oxford : Blackwell, 1976.
2. Ducker TB. Experimental injury of the spinal cord. In: Vinken PJ, Bruya GW, eds. Handbook of clinical neurology Vol. 25. Amsterdam: North Holland Publishing Co. 1976; 9.
3. Michaelis LS. Epidemiology of spinal cord injury. In: Vinken PJ, Bruya GW, eds. Handbook of clinical neurology Vol 35, Amsterdam North Holland Publishing Co., 1976: 141-3.
4. Fine PR, Devivo JM, Mc Eachran AB Re : Incidence of acute traumatic hospitalized spinal cord injury in United States 1970-1977 - letter to the editor. American Journal of Epidemiology 1982; 115: 475-7.
5. Sutton RA, Bently N, Castree B, Mattinson R, Pattinnson J, Smith R. Review of the social situation of paraplegic and tetraplegic patients rehabilitated in Hexham Regional Spinal Injury Unit in the North of England over the past four years. Paraplegia 1982; 20 : 71-9.
6. Masalawala KS. Experience with traumatic paraplegic patients in India. Paraplegia 1975; 13 : 29-35.
7. Braoken MB. Freeman DH, Hallenbrand K. Incidence of acute traumatic hospitalized spinal cord injury in the United States 1970-77. American Journal of Epidemiology, 1981; 113 : 615-22.
8. Rama Rao WG. Needs of a paraplegic in developing countries. Paraplegia 1979; 17: 414.
9. Verma RN, Boparai NS. Paraplegics in the Armed Forces, Medical Journal of the Armed Forces of India 1972; 28 :351-6.
10. Berns SH, Lowman EW, Rusk HA, Covalt DA. Spinal Cord injury - Rehabilitation costs and results of follow up in thirty one cases. Journal of the American Medical Association 1957; 164 : 1551-8.
11. Watson N.A. Survey of non-traumatic paraplegia. Paraplegia 1981; 19: 107-10.
12. Kiwersky J, Chrostowaka T. Social and professional evaluation of para and tetraplegics. Paraplegia, 1982; 20: 97-102.

13. Tarabuloy E. Sexual function in the normal and in paraplegia. Paraplegia 1972; 10 : 201-8.

14. Suri YV. Anaesthetic problems of spinal cord injury patients. Medical Journal of the Armed forces of India 1978; 34 : 374-82.

15. Jellenik HM. Vocational/educational services in medical rehabilitation facility-outcome of spinal cord and brain injured patients. Archieves of physical Medicine and Rehabilitatioin 1982; 63:87.

16. Jenik F, Kuha W, Zach ZA. Social and vocational reintegration of paraplelgic and tetraplegic patients in Switzerland Paraplegia 1982; 20 : 65-70.

17. Samy A. Role of sheltered workshop in the rehabilitation of the physically handicapped. Journal of Rehabilitation in Asia 1980; 21 : 28-31.

Chapter-22

Tobacco Smoking Habits Among Army Personnel in Pune Cantonment

Abstract

Salient findings of study of tobacco smoking habits among army personel in various units of Pune Cantonment have been brought out in his article. Rankwise prevalence and other behavioural aspects have also been highlighted. Findings revealed that greater emphasis on health educational efforts, both at personal and family levels to curb this unhealthy habit of smoking among army personnel, is required.

Introduction

Smoking is probably the largest single preventable cause of ill health today in the world. In many developing countries the epidemic of smoking-related diseases has already assumed a high magnitude which can easily be compared with any infectious diseases or malnutrition, posing as a public health problem. The studies conducted at the Royal College of Physicians revealed that one in three cigarette smokers deaths caused could directly be attributed to the habit of smoking and on an average each cigarette smoked shortens the life of the smokers 5½ minutes[1]. Statistics further showed that 90 per cent of deaths due to cardiovacular diseases and 75 per cent due to chronic bronchitis stem directly from the smoking. The World Health Organization expressed serious concern over smoking and selected a theme as Smoking or Health - the Choice is Yours for WHO Day during 1980.

Several studies have been conducted on various aspects of smoking including school children medical students, doctors relatives and attendants of patients, patients themselves, industrial workers secondary school teachers etc. * However no exhaustive study has been carried out India with * smoking habits of army personnel. Health is of paramount * efficiency of troops while in service and subsequent the * retirement. All efforts in maintaining good health would go * troops fall victims of smoking habits. Therefore, the present study has been undertaken to identity various factors responsible for smoking.

Material and Methods

A representative sample of 400 army personnel serving in various military units of Pune Cantonment was selected out of the total available population following stratified random sampling technique[12].

Findings and Discussion

1. Prevalence of tobacco smoking habit and distribution of smokers and non-smokers according to present age: Out of 400 subjects studied 180 of them were found to be smokers. However, in another study on smoking habits of men in Rajasthan, it was noted that 68.6 per cent of military personnel were smokers[13]. The group-wise age distribution is given in Table 1.

Table 1

Distribution of Smokers and Non-Smokers According to Present Age

S. No.	*Age group (years)*	*Smokers*	*Non-Smokers*	*Total*
1.	15-24	48 (26.66%)	83 (37.73%)	131
2.	25-34	75 (41.67%)	70 (31.82%)	145
3.	35 and above	57 (31.67%)	67 (30.45%)	124
	Total	180 (100.00%)	220 (100.00%)	400

$X^2 = 6.39$; $df = 2$; $p < 0.05$

It is evident that majority of the smokers belonged to the age group of 25-34 years. The difference between this and other age groups was found to be statistically significant (p <0.05). However, these findings of the present one could not be compared with any other study in respect of army personnel due to non-avilability of any published work commenting on this aspect. This finding suggests that there is as greater need to educate this age group about smoking and associated health hazards.

2. Socio-economic status and smoking habit: Already a built-in social classification exists in the form of rank structure in the Army officers, Junior Commissioned Officers (JCOs) and other ranks (OR). The same was utilized as a basis for socio-economic classification of the study population. Distribution of smokers and non-smokers according to rank is presented in Table 2.

Table 2
Distribution of Smokers and Non-Smokers According to Rank

S. No.	*Age group (years)*	*Smokers*	*Non-Smokers*	*Total*
1.	Officers	17 (44.74%)	21 (55.26%)	38
2.	JCOs	18 (45.00%)	22 (55.00%)	40
3.	OR	145 (45.03%)	177 (54.97%)	322
	Total	180	220	400

$X^2 = 0.0012$; df = 2; $p > 0.05$

The table reveals that there was a slightly higher proportion of smokers in other ranks (OR) as compared to JCOs and officers. The prevalence of smoking has not been found to be associated with rank ($p > 0.05$). Authors of other studies with different population groups in UK, however, noticed an increase in smoking habit with decrease in social class[14, 15]. The finding indicates that all army personnel, irrespective of their ranks, need to be covered under a programme of health education on smoking and its health hazards.

3. Family history of smoking: It is evident from Table 3, that more number of smokers confirmed family history of smoking (especially among father and brothers) as compared to non-smokers. The association between smoking in study population and family history was found to be statistically significant ($p < 0.01$). This finding is also in confirmity with the findings of other studies, reporting a higher prevalence of smoking among those who elicted a family history of smoking among parents and/ or siblings[16,17,18]. This implies that besides educating the individual, thee family as a whole must be made the target of our health education, if we want to desist our children from falling prey to this unhealthy habit.

Table 3
Distribution of smokers and non-smokers as per family history of smoking

S. No.	*Family Member**	*Smokers*	*Non-Smokers*	*Total*
1.	Father	104 (57.78%)	89 (40.45%)	193
2.	Mother	7 (3.89%)	3 (1.36%)	10
3.	Brother	77 (42.78%)	48.(21.82%)	125
4.	Sister	1 (0.56%)	- -	1
5.	None	53 (29.44%)	106 (48.18%)	159

* More than one answer was permitted

4. Inducement to smoking by friends: It is seen that 47.22 per cent of smokers were induced by their friends and got into the habit while 29.55 per cent of non-smokers were also induced at one time or the other, but did not fall prey to this habit as shown in Table 4. The inducement was found to be absent in 52.78 per cent of smokers and 70.45 per cent of non-smokers. This difference between smokers and non-smokers in relation to inducement be friends was found to be statistically significant ($p < 0.01$). These findings are similar to those studies in which the friends were found to be thee main instigators in inducing smoking habit in 65 per cent. Such inducement by their smoker friends and-not to be a victim to their tactics and pressure. This caution should form an important ingradicnt of all health education against smoking.

Table 4

Distribution of smokers and non-smokers according to inducement to smoking by friends

S. No.	Inducement by Friends	Smokers	Non-Smokers	Total
1.	Present	85 (47.22%)	65 (29.55%)	150
2.	Absent	95 (52.78%)	155 (70.45%)	250
	Total	180 (100.0%)	220 (100.0%)	400

$X^2 = 13.2$; df =1; $p<0.001$

5. ***Smoking and other addictions:*** The tobacco smoking habit was more prevalent among users of alcohal and other dependence producing drugs such as bhang (cannabis preparation) (Table 5). The association of smoking and other dependence producing drugs was found to be statistically signficant ($p<0.001$). In a survey conducted on rural male population in Punjab, 21.9 per cent alcohol users were found to be addicted to tobacco smoking also[19]. But the present survey in army population has revealed a higher proportion (51.45 per cent) of smokers among alcohol users. There is, thus, a clear cut need for a comprehensive health education programme not only against tobacco smoking but als against alcohol and other addictions as well.

Table 5

Combination of smoking with alcohal and other dependence producing drugs

S.No.	Groups	Number	Alcohol use		Use of drugs	
			Yes	No	Yes	No
1.	Smokers	180	142 (51.45%)	38 (30.65%)	8 (88.89%)	172 (43.99%)
2.	Non-smokers	220	134 (48.55%)	86 (69.35%)	1 (11.11%)	219 (56.01%)
Total		400	276 (100%)	124 (100%)	9 (100%)	391 (100%)

$p< 0.01$

6. Awareness of health hazards of tobacco smoking: It is obvious from Table 6 that a large proportion of both, smokers and non-smokers, were aware of some of the hazards of smoking. The difference in proportions between smokers and non-smokers in relation to such awareness was not statistically significant (p>0,05). Such awareness among smokers is a welcome feature. Further, it must be strengthened by imparting health education repeatedly in various forms to force these people to give up this unhealthy education habit. At the same time awareness will be aroused in those who are still ignorant of the health hazards of tobacco smoking by carrying out vigorous health campaigns as a regular activity.

Table 6

Distribution of smokers and non-smokers as per awareness of specific health hazards of smoking

S.No.	*Specific health hazards**	*Smokers*	*Non-smokers*
1.	Chest disease	157 (87.22%)	165 (75.00%)
2.	Lung cancer	98 (54.44%)	127 (57.33%)
3.	Heart diseases	4 (2.22%)	8 (3.64%)
4.	Abdominal disease	8 (4.44%)	1 (0.45%)
5.	None	12 (6.67%)	10 (4.55%)

*More than one answer was permitted

7. Form of smoking: It is evident that majority of smokers preferred cigarettes. None of the smokers in the present study was found smoking ***hookah, chillum,*** cigar or pipe (Table 7). The findings of present study are similar to those who also reported a higher proportion of cigarette smokers[17, 21], but they differed from some workers[20, 22]. These variations are due to basic differences in the nature of the population studies. However, the point to be emphasised during health education is that whatever may be the form of smoking, it always poses a health hazard and is, therefore, undesirable. Unlike cigarette packets, the other form of smoking may not be carrying a warning, but nonetheless, they are equally harmful.

Table 7

Distribution of Smokers According to form of Smoking

S.No.	*Form of smoking*	*Number*	*Percentage*
1.	Cigarettes	91	50.56
2.	Bidis	45	25.00
3.	Both	44	24.44
	Total	180	100.00

8. Quantity of smoking: According to amount of smoking, the smokers were classified into three categories-mild smokers (less than ten ***bidis*** or cigarettes per day). Moderate smokers (between ten and 20 ***bidis*** or cigarettes per day) and heavy smokers (more than 20 ***bidis*** or cigarettes per day). Their distribution is shown in Table 8.

Table 8

Distribution of Smokers According to Quantity of Smoking

S.No.	*Type of smoker as per quantity*	*Form of smoking*			
		Cigarettes	*Bidis*	*Both*	*Total*
1.	Mild	62 (68.13%)	22 (48.89%)	21 (47.73%)	105 (58.33%)
2.	Moderate	28 (30.77%)	14 (31.11%)	15 (34.09%)	57 (31.67%)
3.	Heavy	1 (1.10%)	9 (20.00%)	8 (18.18%)	18 (10.00%)
	Total	91 (100%)	45 (100%)	44 (100%)	180 (100%)

$X^2 = 10.2$; df = 2; $p < 0.01$

It is seen that majority of smokers were mild smokers irrespective of the form of smoking. A significant relationship was observed between the form of smoking and amount of tobacco smoked by the smokers ($p < 0.01$). These findings are similar to the studies which also reported a preponderance of light smokers [20, 23]. However, as per the findings of survey conducted in Rajasthan revealed military personnel in the age group of heavy smokers (21-25 cigarettes per day)[13]. While imparting health education to the troops they should be informed that although the heavy smokers are exposed to serious health hazards but even mild smokers are also not totally free from it Irrespective of the amount of smoking, it still remains a potential health hazard.

Table 9

Distribution of Smokers and Non-Smokers according to Source of Information on Hazards of Smoking

S.No.	*Source**	*Smokers*	*Non-smokers*
1.	Radio	57 (31.67%)	55 (25.00%)
2.	Doctors/Friends	42 (23.33%)	57 (25.91%)
3.	Warning on cigarettes packets	49 (27.22%)	40 (18.18%)
4.	Own experience	27 (15.55%)	52 23.64%)
5.	Television	41 (22.78%)	33 (15.00%)
6.	Newspapers	34 (22.78%)	23 (10.45%)
7.	Books	17 (9.44%)	17 (7.73%)
8.	Magazines	9 (5.00%)	22 (10.00%)

* More than one answer was permitted.

9. Sources of information on hazards of smoking: Radio, doctors/friends, warning on cigarette packets own experience and television were found to be the main sources of information as shown in Table 9, on hazards of tobacco smoking. The most popular media must continue to be utilised for imparting health education against tobacco smoking but simultaneously other media should also carry messages on this subject more frequently. ***Sainik Samachar,*** Monthly Newsletter (***Baat Cheet***) and regimental corps news bulletins should also be utilised for this purpose.

Acknowledgement

The authors are grateful to the officers commanding various army units in Pune Cantonment for their wholehearted support in providing necessary information and making their personnel available for this study. The authors are also thankful to Shri S.S. Ganguly, Chief Statistician, Armed Forces Medical College, Pune for his guidance on sampling techniques and subsequent statistical analysis.

References

1. Russell, N.A.H. (1981) Excerpts from 'Nicotine Intake and its Regulation', *World Smoking and Health.* 6: (1), p. 34-42.
2. Central Health Education Burau, New Delhi (1980), 'Smoking or Health: The Choice is Yours'. *Swasth Hindi,* p. 24-53.
3. Mahler, H. (1980) 'Smoking or Health: The Choice is Yours'. World Health Day, April 7, (1980) (Editorial). *World Smoking and Health.* 5 (1): 2.
4. World Health Organization (1979) Controlling the Smoking Epidemic *WHO Tech. Rep.* Ser. No. 636.
5. Babu, D.S. & Chuttani, C.S. (1978) Respiratory Symptoms and Smoking among School Children, *Indian J. Prev. Soc. Med.* 9: p 4-7.
6. Roy, M. & Chakraborty, A.K. (1981) Smoking and Drug Abuse among the Newly Admitted Students of Medical Colleges in West Bengal, *Indian J. Public Health,* 25: 30-5.
7. Doll, R. & Hill, A.S. (1964) Mortality in Relation to Smoking: TenYears Observations of British Doctors. *Br. Med. J.:* p. 1399-1410.
8. Vishwanathan, R. (1964) Chronic Bronchitis Emphysema Syndrome Incidence, Aetiology and Natural History. *Indian J. Chest. Dis.* 6: p. 171-182.
9. Brett. G.Z. & Benjamin, B. (1968) Smoking Habits of Men Employed in Industry and Mortality. *Br. Med. J.* 3: 82-5.
10. Thiruvengadam, K.V. Sekar, T.S. & Rajagopal, K.R. (1974) Study of Chronic Bronchitis in Tamil Nadu, *Indian J. Chest. Dis.* 16: p. 1-10.

11. Morries, J.F. & Tichy. M.W. (1970) Smoking Habits and Attitudes of Oregon Secondary School Coaches. *Am. J. Public Health.* 60: p. 1-10.
12. Cochran, W.G. (1967) Sampling Technique, Modern Asia ed. John Wiley and Sons. Inc. New York and Charles E. Tuttle Company, Tokyo. p. 53-54.
13. Brown, A.S., Singh, T.I., Bhown, M. & Maitrya, B.S. (1973) A Survey Report on Smoking Habits of Men in Rajasthan. *J. Indian Med. Assoc.* 60: p. 107-109.
14. Rimington, J. (1969) Chronic Bronchitis, Smoking and Social Class. A Study among Working People in the Towns of Mid and East Cheshire. *Br. J. Chest Dis.* 63: p. 193.
15. Ashwell, M., North, W.R.S. & Meade, T.W. (1978) Social Class, Smoking and Obesity. *Br. Med. J.* 2: p. 1466-1467.
16. Babu, D.S. & Chuttani, C.S. (1977) Some Factors Influencing the Onset of Cigarette Smoking among School Children. *Indian J. Prev. Soc. Med.* 8: p. 71-74.
17. Jindal, S.K., Malik, S.K. & Qamra, S.R. (1982) A Study on the Habits and Attitude Aspects of Tobacco Smoking in Chandigarh. *Indian J. Chest. Dis. Allied Sci.* Special Number, Smoking and Health. p. 14-23.
18. Sandell, J., Singh, S., Sati, T.K. & Mehrotra, S.K. (1983) A Study of Smoking Habits of Medical Students of Uttar Pradesh. *Indian J. Public Health,* 27: p. 96-101.
19. Mohan, D., Sharma, B.K., Sundaran, K.R., & Neki, J.S. (1980) Pattern of Alcohol Consumption of Rural Punjab Males. *Indian J. Med. Res.* 72: p. 702-711.
20. Bhattacharyya, S.N., Bhatnagar, J.K., Kumar, S. & Jain, P.C. (1975) Chronic Bronchittis in Rural Population. *J. Chest. Dis.* 17: p. 1-7.
21. Malik, S.K. (1982) Tobacco Smoking, Product Preference and Chronic Bronchitis. *Indian J. Chest. Dis. Allied Sci.* Special Number: Smoking and Health. p. 83-90.
22. Malik, S.K. & Singh, K. (1978) Smoking Habits, Chronic Bronchitis and Ventilatory Function in Rural Males. *Indian J. Chest. Dis. Allied Sci.* 20: p. 73-9.
23. Wig, K.L., Guleria, J.S., Bhasin, R.C., Holmes, B.J.R., Vasudeva, Y.L. & Singh, H. (1964) Certain Clinical and Epidemiological Aspects of Chronic Bronchitis as seen in Northern India. *Indian J. Chest. Dis.* 6: p. 183-194.

Chapter–23

Psychosocial Profile of Inmates of Orphanages

Abstract

A psychosocial study of 306 institutionalised orphans was carried out at Pune. Various aspects like age, sex, religion-wise distribution including their age at entry, social status of parents and type/cause of destitution have been studied. The intelligence quotient (IQ) and early psychological symptoms of the inmates have also been highlighted.

Introduction

The abandonment of a child is an act of gross violation of human rights. The abandoned child is deprived of a personal and social identity - a big social handicap for his future life. In the absence of timely intervention, abandonment is an immediate threat to the child's survival, protection, care and preparation for life. In turn, this unfortunate individual becomes a burden to society at large. (1)

For years, orphans have been the brunt of cruelty and indifference of adults. Merely making institutions for them is no real solution to the problem. They must have deep human compassion of those who are prepared to give them love and real foundation of individual character and discipline, which can prove to be an incentive for great achievements by the individuals towards society at large. (2)

Institutional care has its short-comings, perhaps not so much the mere absence of maternal and paternal relationship but the ethos of the institution, the demonstration that they are "different" may be the reason for the same. (3)

The Government of India declared a National Policy for Children on August 22, 1974 which lays down a 15-point programme in areas of health, nutrition, education and recreation with five major areas of activity: (a) promotive and preventive aspects of child health; (b) nutrition of infants, pre-school children; (c) maintenance, education and training of orphans and destitute children; (d) day care and other services for children of working mothers; and (e) rehabilitation of handicapped children. (4)

There is marked paucity of available data on the subject of health and nutritional status of children in orphanages. Even in cases where adequate health and nutritive facilities are available, children frequently exhibit "failure to thrive" due to impersonal nature of the care provided. When deprived of parental care, the child's development is likely to be retarded physically, intellectually and socially and symptoms of physical and mental illness may appear. (5, 6)

The present study was undertaken with a view to fill up the gaps in our existing knowledge on the social etiology of destitution as well as to bring out a psychosocial profile of the orphans.

Materials and Method

The study population comprised inmates of the folowing four orphanages :

- i Tyabia Orphanage provided a study population fo 92 orphans in the age group of 5-18 years.
- ii St. John's Orphanage provided a study population of 45 orphans in the age group of 0-5 years.
- iii St. Gabriel's Orphanage provided a study of population of 54 orphans in the age group of 5-10 years.
- iv St. Michael's Orphanage provided a study population of 115 orphans in the age group of 10-18 years.

Thus, the study population consisted of 306 children.

A liaison was established with the governing body, administrators and social workers of these institutions and a plan was also chalked out as per their convenience before the commencement of the study. The data was collected by interviewing the study subjects and by recording on a pretested schedule.

Secondary data was collected from the records maintained at the orphanages in regard to information not readily forthcoming from the individuals, viz., reasons for their entry into the orphanages.

IQ test was carried out for children aged 5-10 years by Draw-a-Man technique. For this, guidance was taken from the Psychiatry Department, Armed Forces Medical College, Pune, while analysing the data. To corroborate the findings the assistance of psychosocial worker was also taken.

Results and Discussion

Age Distribution: The age-wise break up of children in the various orphanages has been studied and shown in Table 1.

Table 1

Age group Years	*St. John*		*St. Gabriel*		*St. Michael*	*Tayabia*	*Total*
0-2	15	10	-	-	-	-	21
2-4	9	7	-	-	-	-	16
4-6	5	3	7	5	-	4	24
6-8	-	-	11	7	-	18	36
8-10	-	-	10	14	-	17	41
10-12	-	-	-	-	26	16	42
12-14	-	-	-	-	33	17	50
14-16	-	-	-	-	36	14	50
16-18	-	-	-	-	20	6	26
Total	29	20	28	26	115	92	306

There were 37 children (9.15%) in the age group 0-4 years as compared to Pathak and Saxens's (1980) estimate of 13.09 percent children in that age group. There were 80 children (26. 14%) in the age group 5-9 years and 113 children (39. 92%) in the age group of 10-14 years. The comparable figures estimated by Pathak and Saxena were 33.57 percent and 53.34 percent respectively. However, their study calculations were based on the figures for children in the age group 0-14 years while this study dealt with the age group of 0-18 years. (7, 8)

The break-up in the present study does not necessarily represent the distribution of orphans in the community as all orphans do not get equal opportunity to join the orphanages.

Sex-wise Distribution: Sex-wise break-up of children has been examined and shown in Table 2.

Table 2

Institution	*Male*	*Female*	*Total*
Tayabia Orphanage	92	-	92
St. John's Orphanage	25	20	45
St. Gabriel's Orphanage	28	26	54
St. Michael's Orphanage	-	115	115
Total	145	161	306

Tayabia orphanage caters only for boys while St. Michael's caters only for girls. There was a total of 145 male orphans (47.39%) and 161 female orphans (52. 61%) which formed the study population.

This may not reveal the true sex-wise distribution of orphans in the community at large as most orphans do not get opportunity for admission to various institutions. Further, a small intake was only possible due to the limited capacity of the institutions.

Religion-wise Distribution: Religion wise distribution of inmates in orphanages were studied and has been shown in Table 3.

Table 3

Religion	*St. John*	*St. Gabriel*	*St. Michael*	*Tayabia*	*Total*
Hindu	26	32	85	-	143
Christianas	18	20	28	-	66
Muslims	1	2	2	92	97
Total	45	54	115	92	306

This religion-wise distribution of orphans does not represent the true picture of orphans in the community. For example, in the present study, Tayabia orphanages was exclusively meant for Muslim inmates while in other orphanages entry of Christian orphans was mostly favoured.

Age at Entry into Orphanages: The average age of entry in the orphanages has been studied (other than Tayabia orphanage where children below five years were not admitted) which was found to be 4.61 years for boys and 3.81 years for the girls. This possibly reflects our social environment in which girls become destitute much earlier. The findings here found to be in conformity with those of Tandon (1981) who observed that parental loss generally occurred before the age of five years.

Table 4

Social Stuatus	*St. John*	*St. Gabriel*	*St. Michael*	*Tayabia*	*Total*
I Professional	-	-	-	-	-
II Semi-Professional	-	-	-	-	-
III Clerical, Office worker	2	4	11	3	20
IV Skilled worker	12	14	25	22	73
V Unskilled worker	13	15	34	27	89
VI Unemployed	6	5	10	7	28
VII Not known	12	16	35	33	96
Total	45	54	115	92	306

Social Status of Parents: As the monthly income of parents of inmates was not mentioned in the records it was extremely difficult to ascertain their social status. Hence, the standard scales for social status could not be applied. An effort was made to assess the social status by means of occupation of the parents as has been shown in Table 4. Even then the occupation of parents could not be found out in respect of 96 children. However, most of the children in the study belonged to the lower social class and were the under privileged members of the society.

Type of destitution: An effort was made to classify orphans on the basis of whether their parents were alive or not. Orphans with no parents alive were classified as complete orphans and with only mother alive as paternal orphans. The type of destitution has been shown in Table 5.

Table 5

Type of Destitute	*St. John*		*St. Gabriel*		*St. Michael*	*Tayabia*	*Total*		*% age*
	M	F	M	F	F	M	M	F	
Complete Orphans	11	15	4	8	37	24	39	60	32.35
Maternal Orphans	6	2	6	5	18	20	32	25	18.63
Paternal Orphans	8	3	18	13	60	48	74	76	49.02
Total	25	20	28	26	115	92	145	161	100.00

The distribution of orphans appears to be at variance with the estimate by Pathank and Saxena (1980). Their estimate was that there were 50.57 percent paternal orphans, 36 percent maternal orphans and 5.07 percent complete orphans. This discrepancy was found because of a tradition in our society that on the death of the head of the family (the father), the mother is incapable of looking after herself and her children. In the present study deserted children without any history were taken as complete orphans and hence were in larger numbers as compared to the findings of Pathak and Saxena's estimates.

A glaring reflection of our socio-cultural milieu is the fact that out of 99 complete orphans, 60 were females.

Causes of Destitution: The causes of destitution in respect of orphans have been given in Table 6.

Table 6

Causes	*St. John*	*St. Gabriel*	*St. Michael*	*Tayabia*	*Total*
Complete Orphans					
Found on street	16	3	12	16	47
Immoral danger	7	5	10	3	25
Unmarried mothers	-	-	5	-	5
Parent beggars	1	2	3	-	6
Information was not available	1	3	7	5	16
Maternal Orphans					
Complication of pregnancy	4	1	6	4	15
Miscellaneous disease	3	3	1	4	11
Unknown cause	1	7	11	12	31
Paternal Orphans					
Old age	-	1	9	6	16
Chronic alcoholism	3	2	3	5	13
Miscellaneous disease	5	8	10	6	29
Unknown cause	3	20	38	31	92
Total	44	55	115	92	306

(df = 8; $p < 0.05$; X = 5.388)

Relevant information was not forthcoming in respect of 54.58 percent of cases as is evident from Table 6. This was possibly due to the fact that orphans were generally deserted and hence unable to provide the required information. In view of the above facts the data was not considered adequate for applying the tests of significance for the total study population. However, Chi Square test was carried out on the information available (i.e. 45.42%) and yet the difference between the information available in the orphanages of the present study was not found to be significant.

While reviewing the literature, although the breakups of paternal, maternal and complete orphans are mentioned, further break-down of causes of death/desertion are not highlighted. As such, these have not been attempted here.

Intelligence Quotient: Distribution of orphans as per their IQ has been given in Table 7.

Table 7

IQ		*Tayabia*	*St. Gabriel*	*Total*	*Percentage*
Idiot	0-24	-	-	-	-
Imbecile	25-49	-	-	-	-
Moron	50-69	1	1	2	2.15
Border-line	70-79	9	10	19	20.43
Low-normal	80-89	15	29	44	47.31
Normal	90-109	12	12	24	25.81
Superior	110-119	1	1	2	2.15
Very superior	120-139	1	1	2	2.15
Near genius	140	-	-	-	-
Total		39	54	93	100.00

Note: Only children aged 5-10 years were considered for study.

(df = 2; X^2 = 2.388; p > 0.05)

As mentioned earlier, IQ was worked out by Draw-a-man test for orphans between the ages of 5-10 years. Out of 93 children examined, two children were morons (2.15%), 19 children had borderline, 24 children had normal IQ (25.81%), two children had superior IQ (2.15%), while two children had very superior IQ (2.15%). The difference in IQ between the two orphanages was not found to be significant. Hence, it was inferred that IQ of orphans, given a healthy environment, was adequate.

These findings were at complete variance with Wolkund's observation of IQ 50-70 (morons) in 40.3 percent children in Indian orphanages. (10)

The most common group in the present study was low normal IQ (IQ 80-90) in which 47.31 percent of the children were placed. Whether this had any correlation with destitutioin is at present a matter of conjecture and would require a more detailed study.

Early Psychological Symptoms: Early psychological symptoms among residents studied in the orphanages were shown in Table 8.

Table 8

Sr. No	*Symptoms*	*Complete orphan*	*Maternal orphan*	*Paternal orphan*	*Total*
1.	Demands attention	38	15	5	58
2.	Nail biting	20	10	3	33
3.	Defiances	13	4	5	22
4.	Stammering	2	1	0	3
5.	Excessive temper	11	2	1	14
6.	Vomitting bouts	9	3	1	13
7.	Excessively violent	7	2	3	12
8.	Truancy	2	6	4	12
9.	Excessive nervousness	5	3	2	10
10.	Nightmares	2	1	-	3
11.	Subnormal mental growth	2	1	-	3
12.	Bed-wetting	6	3	1	10
13.	Backwardness in school	4	1	1	6
	Total	121	52	26	199

Note: 261 children in age group of 5-18 years were examined. 199 symptoms were found in 111 children.

(df = X^2 + 9.734; $p > 0.05$)

Early psychological manifestations were looked for in the age group 5-18 years and 111 children of the study subjects (42.52%) were found to have these symptoms. Some children had more than one psychological problems.

These symptoms were encountered much more in complete orphans. 64 out of 73 complete (87.67%), 31 out of 49 maternal (63.26%) and 16 out of 139 paternal orphans (11.51%) had early psychological manifestations. There was a significant difference in the number of complete and maternal orphans having early psychological symptoms as compared to paternal orphans. The average number of symptoms was 1.89, 1.67 and 1.62 in each affected complete, maternal and paternal orphans respectively. There was no significant difference in the type of early psychological symptoms between these three groups.

The findings of the study revealed that the loss of the mother in early childhood had telling effects on the individual's psyche. It also brought out that the complete orphan was under severe stress which could affect adversely on his psychological well-being later in life.

Further, no child was found with stealing habit. This was possibly due to good institutional guidance. The other findings were similar to the observations made by Wolkund (10) who found that the four most common psychiatric problems among orphans were quarrelsome nature, destructive behaviour, bedwetting and stealing.

In the present study the more common symptoms were found among complete orphans and maternal orphans. This is in conformity with the findings of Burlingham (11) who had noted a special relationship between early psychological symptoms and maternal loss. Stein (12) had also observed that persistent bedwetting seemed to be connected with disturbance in child's relation with the mother.

In conclusion, the institutionalised orphans in the study population generally belonged to lower social strata of society, entered the orphanage before the age of five years, suffered from early psychological problems and had lower IQ than the general population. It also indicatd that periodical psychological assessment and psychotherapy may be necessary for an orphan before he leaves the institution.

Reference

1. UNICEF (1984) The Destitute Child 12, (2).
2. Brown. F. (1966) Child Bereavement and Subsequent Psychiatric Disorders. Brit. J. Psych. 118, p. 319-27.
3. Koller, K.M. (1971) Paternal Deprivation, Family Background and Female Delinquency. Brit. J. Psych. 118, p. 319-27.

4. National Institute of Social Defence (1982) Operating Manual for Children Act, 1982, 14.

5. Rane, Asha (1986) Children in Difficult Situations - A Review. Tata Institute of Social Sciences, p. 2-15 241.

6. Athala, Usha (1986) Inadequacies in Institutionalised Infant Care (Mimeo).

7. Lotka, A.J. (1931) Orphanhood in Relation to Demographic Factors-A Study of Population Analysis Matron. IX, (2), p. 37-109.

8. Tandon, A.K. & Tandon, R.K. (1981) Parental Deprivation and Delinquency. Ind Paed. SV (1), p. 33.

9. Pathak B. & Saxena A. (1980) Revised Estimates of Orphans and Probability of Orphanhood.

10. Wolkund S. (1980) Psychiatric Morbidity in Children Homes, Indian J. Psych. P. 236.

11. Burlingham. Freod (1944) Infants Without Families. Allen and Unurn, London.

12. Stein, Z. & Susser M.W. (1965) Socio-medical Study of Enuresis Among Delinquent Boys. Brit. J. Prev. Soc. Med. 19, p. 174-81.

Chapter–24

Psychosocial Profile of Orphans - An Overview

Introduction

Child is a precious possession of human life in any country and loss of parent in early childhood is one of the greater tragedy of human life. The abandonment of a child is an act of gross violation of human right. The abandoned child is deprived of a personal and social identity-a big social handicap in his future life. In the absence of timely intervention, abandonment is an immediate threat to the child's survival, protection, care and preparation for life. The same also holds good in respect of an orphaned child. (UNICEF 1934) (1).

An average child is tough and resilient and can hope with a personal calamity such as death of a parent, if adequate care is provided. Therefore, the prognosis of an orphaned child largely depends on the efficiency of care provided by an extended family, humane outlook, social services and kindness of neighbours, although these too vary at different places and at different times. That in some cases these factors can prove to be an immense incentive for great achievement is amply evident in case of some poets, writers and other persons of eminence in all walks of life who become orphaned in their early childhood (Brown 1966) (2).

The national policy proclaimed for children on 22 Aug 1974 lays down the following five areas of activity.

(a) Promotive and preventive aspects of child health.

(b) Nutrition of infants, preschool children, nursing and expectant mothers.

(c) Maintenance, education and training of orphans and destitute children.

(d) Day and other services for children of working mother.

(e) Rehabilitation of handicapped children. (3)

There is marked paucity of available literature on the subject of health and nutritional status of children in institutions. Even in cases where adquate health and nutritive facilities are available, children frequently exhibit failure to thrive' due to impersonal nature of the care provided. When deprived of parental care, the child's development is likely to be retarded physically, intellectually and socially and symptoms of physical and mental illness may appear (4).

Classification of Children in difficult situations

Children deprived of adequate care and protection have been classified by Rane (1986) as follows:

A. Juvenile

B. Non delinquents

1. Destitutes

(a) Orphaned

(b) Abandoned

2. Neglected Children

(a) Parents lack economic means

(b) Parents have physical/mental handicap/illness

(c) Children in single parent families

(d) Children of working mother in lower income group

3. Victimised Children

(a) Child beggars

(b) Abused children

(c) Children of prostitutes

(d) Vagrant children

(e) Child workers

(f) Children of parents involved in anti-social activities.

(g) Street children

Table 1
Estimated Number of Destitute Orphan Children in India in 1981 and 1991

Age & Type of orphan	*Estimated number of orphan in hundred* 1981		1991	
	Total	*Destitute*	*Total*	*Destitute*
0-4				
Paternal	21990	8796	16371	6628
Maternal	18182	7273	13856	5543
Complete	428	171	236	94
	40600	16240	30663	12265
5-9				
Paternal	60284	24114	47807	19123
Maternal	54034	21613	43485	17394
Complete	3674	1470	2288	915
	117992	47197	93580	37432
10-14				
Paternal	108347	43339	93221	37288
Maternal	96343	38537	81937	32776
Complete	12640	5056	8603	3441
	217330	85932	183761	73504
Grand Total	375922	105359	308004	123201

Source: Pathak and Saxena (Revised Estimates 1980)

Magnitude of Problem

The working group on Policy and Programmes for Destitute Children (1975) set up by the Planning Commission estimated that 0.5 percent of all children in the age group 0-14 years are destitute (5).

Sushil Chandra in his studies in 1971 in Kanpur reported that 39.72 percent of the destitute had both parents alive, 29 percent had only mother alive, 13.43 percent had only father alive and 13.5 percent had lost both parents (6).

With the help of guidelines provided by the study carrried out by Lotka (1931), Pathak and Saxena (1980) of the International Institute of Population Sciences estimated that in 1971 there were 28.06 millions orphans in age group 0-14 years in India. Of these 19.24 million were paternal orphans, 16.88 million were maternal orphans and 1.92 million were complete orphans (7, 8).

Estimated number of orphans in India in 1981 & 1991 is depicted in Table 1.

Causes of Destitution

Rane etal (1986) stated that deprivations are either economic, social, familial or emotional. The significant factors resulting in deprivation of adequate care and protection are:-

(a) Natural calamities like war, floods, famine, earthquake etc.

(b) Death of one or both parents.

(c) Desertion by either or both parents.

(d) Child birth cut of illegitimate wedlock.

(e) Inability or parents to provide for child care due to extreme poverty.

(f) Physical/mental handicap of one or both parents.

(g) Chronic physical/mental illness of one or both parents.

(h) Family disharmony or marital discord.

(i) Parents' involvement in anti-social activities.

(j) Cruelty of parents/forcing the child to beg or to take to some anti-social activities. (4)

Medical Facilities

There can be no doubt about the fact that medical facilities should exist with every institution holding orphan or destitute children.

The proportion of institutions having medical facilities according to different studies but the highest proportion was 60 percent in a study by Central Social Welfare Board in 1974. This is unfortunately far below the desired level (9).

Rane (1986) observed that even if medical care is provided by the Institution, it's quality is questionable (4).

MORBIDITY SURVEYS: Athale (1979) brings out the inadequacies of institutionalised child care by a study conducted in Bombay. She has concluded that the higher morbidity rate is related to the damage already done before the child is admitted to an institution. (10)

According to Anand (1980) who carried out a study of institutionalised children including infants the infant mortality rates tend to be alarmingly high in institutions. Health and nutritional status of abandoned and destitute children associated with the process of abandonment and destitution as well as quality of institutional services (11).

Gupta (1982) observed that children in orphanage had a lower level personal hygience., low intelligence and tended to have problematic behaviours (12).

HEIGHT AND WEIGHT: Mruthyunjaya (1975) reported that infants who failed to thrive in absence of organic diseases were generally those who had a prolonged separation from their mothers. (12)

Psychological Aspects

For years orphans/destitutes have borne the brunt of cruelty and indifference of society. Merely making institutions for them is no real solution to their problems. Institutions must have deep human compassion of those who are prepared to give them love and real foundation of individual character and discipline. Howard (1944) was of the opinion that even with the best medical set up, it was not possible for any institution to give such children (particularly those of the age group of 0-3 years) the same amount of continuous loving care which a child received from parents (12).

Numerous studies carried out earlier correlates destitution with delinquency. Tandon (1981) in his study at Lucknow found a significantly higher percentage of delinquents belonging to the deprived group (15). Brown (1956) found that paternal and maternal loss responsible for orphanhood are significant factors in both male and female criminality but more marked in female criminality (2), Hill (1967) observed that most of the patients suffering from depression had lost their father before their 15th birthday (16). According to Munro (1965), parental bereavement must always lead to some psychological adverse effect on the child and sometimes this effect may be overwhelming. He concluded that there is little doubt that disturbances in early upbringing always predispose to such abnormalities as psychopathy, delinquency and suicidal tendencies (17).

Wolkund (1980) in his study of Indian orphanages found that the absence of natural parents is the chief characteristic of inmates of orphanages and various kinds of psychiatric disturbances are frequent in such a setting. He further states that no comprehensive study has so far been carried out in respect of orphans in India although thousands of children spend the better part of their life in these institutions (18). He observed that the four most comon psychiatric problems among orphans were stealing, quarrelsome behaviour, destructive behaviour and bed wetting. No significant correlation was found between psychiatric illness, present age, duration of stay and age at entry into orphanages. He also found mild mental retardation (10-50-70) in 40.3 percent of children (18).

Burlingham (1944) observed that there was a special relation between enuresi and maternal loss. Stein (1955) observing that persistent bedwetting seems to be connected with disturbance in child's relationship with mother (19).

Suggestive Corrective Measures

The following corrective measures would alleviate the sufferings of orphans to a great extent:-

(a) Orphans can be looked after better by improving legislation on adoption and encouraging foster care and adoption. This would provide a home to this deprived lot.

(b) On the same lines institutional and uninstitutional sponsorship needs to be increased and facilitated. This can be done by providing incentives for sponsorship.

(c) It is also essential to improve and increase services for one parent orphans e.g. day care services, creches etc.

(d) Welfare services for working children need to improve and be increased by means of improving implementation of existing legislation.

(e) For those orphans who are unable to stay on the 'straight path', the number of juvenile guidance centres and service bureaus needs to be substantially increased.

(f) So as to ensure that others do not join the path of their wayward compatriots it is essential that a thrust be given to the scheme for control and eradication of juvenile begging and vagrancy 1963.

(g) Those orphans who are fortunate to be placed in orphanage also face problems which can be minimised by the following measures:-

   (i) Sufficient trained staff need to be recruited at each orphanage so that adequate care is provided to inmates.

   (ii) Medical facilities including doctor, nurse and sick room should be provided at each orphanage. Regular health appraisal by doctor and staff of the orphanage should be carried out. Maintenance of health record should be compulsory.

(iii) More attention needs to be paid to health education of orphans as well as staff of the orphanage. Personalised care to orphans should be improved so as to reduce disease due to poor personal hygiene as well as early psychological problems.

Reference

1. UNICEF. The Destitute child, 1984 Vol 12, voz
2. Brown. F. Childwood Bereanement and Subsequent Psychiatric Disorders. But. J Psych. 1966 : 112 : 1035-41
3. National Institute of Social-defence. Social defence 1982 X VIII, No 69.
4. Rane Asha. Children in difficult situations - a review. Tata Institute of Social Services; 1986: 2-15, 241
5. National Institute of Public Co-operation and Child Development National Seminar on employment, 1975.
6. Sushil Chandra. Truancy and basic primary education, Indian J Soc Def 1959 Vol 1: 17-31.
7. Lotka A.J. Orphanhood in relation to demographic factor, Matron 1931: Vol IX (2) : 37-109
8. Pathak B. Saxena. A Revised estimates of orphans and probability of orphanhood 1980
9. Central Social Welfare Board, Evaluation and Statistic research Orphanages of India 1974.
10. Athale Usha. Inadequecies in institutionalised infact care. Terres Des Hames India Programme (Mimeo) 1979.
11. Anand RK. Health and Nutritional problems of children in Institutions-paper presented at UNICEF staff orientetion programme 1984.
12. Gupta T. Health of deprived child - study of Orphanages of Lucknow 1982 (unpublished).
13. Mrithyunjaya A. Bansal R.W. Human maternal attachment. Indian Paed 1975 Vol XII No 12: 1233.
14. Howard WH. Institutions serving children 1944-44.

15. Tandon AK. Tandon RK. Parental deprivation and Delinquency, Indian Paed 1981 Vol XV No 1: 33.

16. Hill OW, Pride JC: Childhood bereavement and adult depression. Brit J Psych 1967 : 113 : 743-51.

17. Munro A. Orphanhood and psychiatric diseases. Brit J. Prev and Soc Med 1965 19 : 69-70

18. Wolkund S. Psychiatric morbidity in children homes, Indian J. Psych 1980-236.

19. Burlingham A, Freod, Infants without families, Allen & Unvin London 1944.

Chapter–25

Woman to Woman Education in Delivery of "Non-Formal" Health Care - A New Experience

Abstract

A novel method of woman to woman education for health and delivery was implemented in Maharshtra. The expansion of the new ıntervention including teaching infant feeding practices, various ways of health and nutrition education through this method has been committed in the community.

Introduction

Women play an important role in the health care delivery system, both within and outside the family and also for the community at large. Nevertheless in many instances women do not have the opportunity to realise it because the value of their contribution is always not recognised (1.2). On the contrary, many a times, women were and still are viewed as sources of health problems which require special attention mainly through programmes on maternal and child care, family planning and nutrition.

Of late, women's movements and organizations have been able to reveal their true potential as providers of health care. A fact which is gaining importance now is that when women act as good communicators and motivators for other ladies in the same community in the delivery of health care, the acceptance and practice towards the promotion of a healthy living is far better. Thus, women can play pivotal role in bringing about the positive changes in the women's health status and also in various other aspects of their life styles.

Appreciating this, a research project at a microlevel i.e. at a village level i.e. Malkapur was undertaken by the staff of Dept. of PSM, Krishna Institute of Medical Sciences, Karad. The womenfolk of the study village were educated and motivated to disseminate health messages from woman to woman for improvement of health knowledge. The group, consisting of illiterate, semileterate and educated women was utilised in rendering non formal health care for the benefit of families and for the overall development of the community. Thus, the sources of problems i.e. women were utilised as key resource persons for attaining the goal of 'Health for all by 2000 A.D.'.

Material & Method:

The village Malkapur is situated on the southern outskirts of Karad, in Maharashtra. National Highway No. 4 traverses the village connecting Malkapur with major towns and cities of Western Maharashtra. Out of the three parts of the village viz., Malkapur proper, Shastrinagar and Agashinagar, Malkapur proper was selected for this project as this part represents rural India both socially and culturally.

In early February, 1988, a team was organised, comprising of under graduate medical students, interns and medicosocial workers who were oriented and trained for the project in three successive sessions, each lasting an hour. Subsequently, a meeting was held with the local leaders from the village to explain the purpose of the project and to secure their assistance and co-operation as and when required during the study period. Soon after a public meeting was arranged in the village, primarily involving the women folk of the village. This programme was arranged with defined objectives viz., to explain the objectives of the project to them, to ensure their active involvement and to inspire women to volunteer for the project.

House to house survey was undertaken and data was recorded on a pretested schedule. The survey was undertaken with twin objectives.

(1) To ascertain and analyse the representation of women in the demographic and socio-cultural structure of the village.

(2) To identify the areas requiring intervention, 21 women extended their whole-hearted co-operation and expressed their willingness to participate in the project. A 'Bhagini Mandal' was also formed consisting of these women volunteers as honorary members of the team.

Observation:

Demographic & Socio-cultural profile of women:

Of the 1337 study subjects, 633 were female between 16 and 55 years of age (53.33%) and those above 55 years comprised 7.4 percent. The mean age of the female population was found to be 24.95 years. This indicated that the female population is relatively young and hence amenable to changes towards healthy living.

Literacy rate among female population had improved during the last decade from 7 percent (obtained from Gram Panchayat records) to 53.43 percent. Of these 12 percent could complete middle school education and achieved higher education. Better educational facilities in terms of more number of schools and an independent school for girls, raised socio economic status of individual families and an awareness regarding educatioin among the people were found to be the outstanding reasons for the high female literacy rate in the study village.

Forty two percent of the female villagers were engaged in various occupation, like agriculture, landless labourers, construction and service mainly at Krishna Institute of Medical Sciences and affiliated Hospital and Medical Research Centre,

Malkapur. Of these 19 percent worked in the farms belonging to their families and were not regular employees. The single role ideology was seen in the remaining 58 percent who utilized their time in carrying out household chores.

Conforming, Prasad's classification of social and economic classes in India (1969) and corresponding classifications revised from Gross National Product (1984-85) (1), 54% of the families belonged to Class I and II, 18% to class IV and V and Class III accounted for 28 percent. This clearly indicated that the economy of the surveyed village is reverse to that found in most parts of rural India.

Prevalent cultural practices relevant to health were the age old custom of depriving new born babies of colostrum believing that it is poisonous or hard to digest and simply harmful and should be discarded. Most of the respondents also believed that papaya is an abortificient and is forbidden during pregnancy. Breast feeding was universally accepted and continued for the period varying between 18 months to 3 years. 86 percent of the mothers introduced supplementary food from 6 months onwards while for the remaining infants' weaning commenced very late. Though not common, but one of the popular supplementary foods was the various commercially available baby foods. It was surprising to note that offering "baby foods" was considered as a sign of sound economic status but it was found that these were being offered to infants without following the proper instructions regarding their preparation i.e. these were being given in much diluted forms a cause of subsequent malnutrition. Other supplementary foods included diluted buffalo milk, banana, rice, wheat, chapati, jowar roti, Dal (popularly known as Kalwan) and biscuits. However, the quality and quantity of supplementary foods were found to be poor and inadequate.

These erroneous feeding practices, due to ignorance, misconceptions and traditional beliefs, accounted for the widespread malnutrition present in the under fives which was detected from the anthropometric measurements. Thus, despite, sound economic status and high literacy rate of population, malnutrition was found quite common among the pre-school children-not due to poverty and non-availability of food- but due to "starvation in the midst of plenty"!

Overall lack of awareness regarding personal hygiene was observed particularly amongst women and children.

Areas of Intervention:

After analysing the date collected, areas requiring immediate intervention through Bhagini Mandal, were identified. These included infant feeding, explaining importance of colostrum, personal hygience (particularly of paring off nails and keeping them clean), washing of hands before cooking and consuming correct food, good oral hygiene and nutrition.

Participation solve their own health problem:

To tackle these areas, through an educational approach, 16 sessions, each lasting for 2 to 2½ hours were conducted with help from the members of Bhagini Mandal since December, 1988. The first of these three meetings were utilized to ascertain the level of understanding of the members and to remove communication gaps of language and status and thereby to prepare a ground for subsequent training.

During the remaining sessions, knowledge on the importance of colostrum, infact feeding practices and personal hygience on a scientific basis was imparted. Different methods of communication such as films, flash cards, charts, lectures, demonstrations and role playing were employed for an effective training measure of the group each time. In turn, these women disseminated the information to other women of the village on various occasions e.g. on their work in the filed, visits to temple, public well, flour mills, at social gatherings and their routine visits to the neighbouring house for preparing spices and preservatives, etc.

Four follow-up visits were paid by the team members, every fortnight on completion of the 6th, 9th, 12th & 16th sessions. About 30 percent of the houses were selected randomly for the follow-up.

During follow-up visits, an improvement in the standard of personal hygiene (cutting of nails, washing of hands before cooking and eating, better dental hygiene) was observed in respect of 11 percent of the families.While 29 percent of the women informed about implementing the advice suggested to them on infant feeding, enquiries were made in detail regarding the quantity and quality of foods to be given and the age at which weaning goods were to be started.

This opportunity was also utilised to improve their knowledge on the same subjects on which they were educated and to encourage the further to practice it. The practice of feeding colostrum to the newborn, has been observed in one mother only.

Thus, achievements of our preliminary communications are inspiring and hereafter we intend to cover other important areas also such as age at marriage, family planning, cleanliness in and around the houses etc. for the same community and similar projects on a larger scale for other communities as well in future.

Refrence

1. Chandra, J & Ahmed, S.H. Prasad's Serial Classification of Indian Families: updated. Indian Paidiatrics. 1987, 24 (8) : 689-690
2. Pizurki, H. et at, Women as Providers of Health Cen. Switzerland 1987.
3. Somaiya, P.A. et al. Community Oriented Primary Care. Pritisengam Press, Karad (India), 1988.

Chapter–26

Scope of Health Systems Research in Child Survival and Safe Motherhood Programme

In any community mothers and children constitute a 'priority' group and they comprise approximately 65 per cent of the total-population. By virtue of their sheer numbers, they happen to be the major consumers of the health services. They are also vulnerable to various disease conditions and form risk group. Moreover most of the illnesses and deaths among mothers and children, to a great extent, are preventable (1).

As per recent health statistics (1990) in India, both maternal motality rate (MMR - 5/1000 live births) and infant motality rate (IMR - 80/1000 live births) continue to be high. Few scientific studies conducted earlier revealed that MCH services suffered serious setbacks in India and some of the causes attributed were insufficient planning, lack of manpower, inadequate training and supervision of paramedical personnel, poor utilisation and lack of knowledge among beneficiaries, belief on traditional remedies, low female literacy, inadequate interpersonal communication and information, socio-economic and environmental constraints, lack of epidemiological approach and management skills and ineffective health information system (2).

Analysis of health statistics also revealed that four states of Bihar, Uttar Pradesh, Rajasthan and Madhya Pradesh which constitute about 40 percent of India's population, have IMR and MMR level distinctly higher than the national average (3). These are the states where age at marriage, female literacy status and share of women in non agricultural employment are also distinctly lower than the national average. A further analysis of demographic indicators at district level indicates that there are ninety percent 'below average' districts where even crude birth rate (CBR) is above 39 per thousand, besides high IMR and MMR (4).

Keeping in view the 'Health for All' goal by 2000AD, recently a Child Survival and Safe Motherhood (CSSM) programme has been launched in India with IDA/UNICEF assistance in a phased manner. This programme aims at universalisation of immunisation, diarrhoeal diseases and acute respiratory infection (ARI) control, Vitamin A prophylaxis and new born care. It will also promote safe motherhood through strengthening of antenatal care, iron and folic acid (IFA) supplementation, birth spacing programme and small family norm; and development of improved systems for identification, referral and treatment of obstetric complications. (4)

Main objective of CSSM programme is to reduce the MMR to below 2, IMR to below 50 per thousand and child mortality (1-4) to less than 10 by 2000 AD through improved and expanded MCH services at village, subcentre, primary health centre and community health centre levels. Other activities include improved support system through better training of paraprofessionals, improved logistics support and communication system and better monitoring and evaluation of the existing services. Goals of CSSM also aim at eradication of Poliomyetitis by 2000 AD, elimination of neonatal Tetanus by 1995 and prevention of deaths and cases from measles, diarrrhoeal diseases and acute respiratory infection (pneumonia). (2, 4).

As per Govt. of India policy, all the work related to CSSM would be carried out by existing staff only. This is primarily to rationalise and operationalise the existing job of health functionaries. However supportive services e.g. training, supervision, logistics etc. will be the key strategy for the future success of this project. Similarly IEC (information, education and communication) inputs will have to be revitalised to propagate MCH activities so as to bring attitudinal changes among beneficiaries, specially in rural areas and urban slums.

Health System Research (HSR) is a wide canvas which looks into operationalisation of the health system from policy framing to ultimately making health services available and accessible. The efficacy of HSR as an important tool in health care management has been widely appreciated during last few years and has led to a better understanding of health problems, more rational health policy and programme planning and more effective and efficient use of resources with special reference to primary health care (5).

Primarily HSR aims at developing the health situation, delineating the health policy and improving the operational aspects of health care system and is probably best suported and sustained at district level. HSR, thus, can be regarded as a generic term that includes all types of researches and contributes towards improvement of functioning of health services through providing new information on decision making, supplementing advocacy for introducing changes in health care delivery and contributing to the body of knowledge relating to theories, concepts and methods that would be useful for generating additional information for decision making, supplementing advocacy for introducing changes in health care delivery and contributing to the body of knowledge relating to theories, concepts and methods that would be useful for generating additional information for decision making or providing alternative solution. A symposium in Altermative Strategies in Health Services Research held at Hyderabad sometime ago focussed on the above issues for the first time. (5, 6).

According to some, HSR also attempts to focus on priorities, initiate action plan, to study cost effectiveness and bring out practical and timely solution. Thus it is ultimately concerned with improving the health of a community by enhancing effectiveness and efficiency of health system. (7, 8, 9).

Several multicentric studies have indicated that coverage and quality of MCH services are not upto mark. Some of the underlying causes for the poor perfomance of MCH services have already been mentioned earlier. Considering these aspects, National Institute of Health and Family Welfare (NIHFW) initiated a HSR project with a view to strengthen family welfare (FW) and MCH services including nutrition and school health in Gwalior district for a 5 year period i.e. 1991-95. During 5 years of this District Health Administrative Research (DHAR) project by NIHFW, will be implemented under diagnostic and intervention phase along with continuous monitoring and evaluation using specific MCH indicators, In another ongoing HSR project by Indian Council of Medical Research (ICMR) in this area is directed towards quality assessment of MCH care at PHC level; it's improvement in coverage and quality using "at risk" approach implemented through existing health infrastructure,. It also aims at improving community awareness along with utilisation of MCH services. Even identification of risk factors related to pregnancy outcome has also led to few intervention studies utilising this knowledge. (5, 6, 7).

National evaluation of MCH and FW services at primary health centre was also undertaken by ICMR as a multicentric study. Few evaluation studies, viz. evaluation of anaemia prophylaxis programme, Dai training programme and evaluation of teaching FW & MCH in medical colleges were conducted by NIHFW in the recent past. (8).

Similarly a HSR study of risk approach and intervention strategy in MCH care was undertaken by BJ Medical College, Pune which had on initial phase for identfication of 'at risk' mothers followed by certain interventions through existing peripheral health functioneries with a supporting referral system. It finally evaluated the effectiveness of intervention by demonstrating substantial reduction in perinatal and infant mortality rates ir study area (7, 8).

Health Behaviour Research (HBR) is a part of HSR in its scope and purpose. The primary goal of HBR is an ethical one i.e. to promote participatory health development.

Another aim of HBR is to demystify knowledge and provide means by which decision makers can anticipate, predicat and influence behaviour in order to promote positive health behaviour. Another aim of health behaviour research is to demystify knowledge and provide means by which decision makers can anticipate, predict and influence in order to promote positive health behaviour (10).

If the technology available in modern medicine is to reach the majority of the 'vulnerable' group, considerable changes in health behaviour are needed, yet this information as to how to achieve the same is inadequate. It is now acknowledged by research workers as well as health administrators that social sciences research is indicated in order to understand the origin and problems faced within MCH services. Though some attention has been paid by few social scientists to the malnutrition problems among pregnant mothers and under 5 children, yet the incidence of low birth weight (LBW) babies and to the deteoriation of women's health, but it is now realised that many other socio-cultural and economic issues are also involved. (10).

To cite common examples, some research workers have observed that in many households where food is available, unequal social status between men and women have resulted in unequal feeding i.e. women eat only whatever is left over after feeding the rest of family members. Similarly some taboos and distinction between 'hot' and 'cold' foods and vegetarians are occasional subjects of malnutrition. These aspects need to be studied under health behavioural research (8, 10).

Underutilisation of health services specially by pregnant mothers and under 5 children is another high priority area for further research. One of the objectives would be to ascertain how MCH services can accommodate the indigenous health system of which child birth is a part and can strengthen woman's participation in order to improve health education programme. Similarly, although training of trained birth attendants can improve the linkage between home-centred system and MCH services, it may fail if the back up primary health care (PHC) system has no understanding of local health culture. (10).

These are few examples which have been discussed in brief and there are many more grey areas' for application of HSR in the field of MCH.

From this above discussion, few key issues emerge. Regarding application of HSR for improvement of mother and child care. Though few epidemiological studies-both diagnostic and evaluation were undertaken by ICMR, NIHFW and handful of research workers during last few years, but it is reiterated that there is wide scope for application of HSR for further improvement and bringing out some alternative models in MCH services. It is felt that this sensitive and important discipline did not receive its due attention that it deserves from research workers and specialists practicing in this field. Even there is a large gap between planning of MCH services and it's implementation in the field-right from national to grassroot level.

Analytical and intervention research studies are not many and hardly any research studies based on modern managements technique e.g. operational research (OR) or systems analysis have been undertaken applying the principles of HSR including HBR (10).

One can only hope and look forward with optimism that some research institutions workers would come forward with new ideas to broaden their professional horizon and apply the principles of OR or Systems analysis in CSSM programme. It is needless to say such study should be holistic and involve a multidisciplinary team work i.e. specialists from the disciplines of obstetrics, paediatrics, epidemiology, health administration, social scientists drawn from medical sociology, medical anthropology, economics etc, who can design an indepth study for improvement of CSSM programme. In this regard, it may also be mentioned that before and during conducting such diagnostic/intervention/evaluation studies, important key persons like policy makers, political decision makers, peoples' representatives and senior administrators should also be sensitised/involved to apply the potential of HSR in the field of MCH for improving the overall functioning of the CSSM programme. (11).

References

1. Park's Text Book of Preventive and Social Medicine J. E. Park & K. Park, 13th Edition, Dec. 19991. M/s. Banarsidas Bhanot. Jabalbur, Pg. 299.
2. Guidelines on National Child Survival and Safe Motherhood Programme - Deptt. of Family Welfare, Min. of Health & Family Welfare, Govt. of India, New Delhi. 1992 (Minlographed) Pg. 1-4.
3. Annual Report 1991-92 Ministry of Health & Family Welfare, Government of India. Pg. iv), 27-32.
4. The Journal of Family Welfare, Vol. 38, No. 3, September, 1992 Special Issue, 40 years of IPPF, 1952-19992, Family Planning Association of India, Bombay Pg. 61.
5. National Conference of Health Systems Research - Introductory Document National Institute of Health & Family Welfare, New Delhi Pg. 13-15.
6. District Health Systems Research Projects in Gwalior MP (1991-95) National Institute of Health & Family Welfare, New Delhi Pg. 13-15.
7. National Conference on Health Systems Research, NIHFW 14-18 December, 1992, Inaugural Address by Dr. V. Ko Ko Regional Director, WHO South East Asia Region pg. 2-4.
8. Health services/Systems Research under this Auspices of The Indian Council of Medical Research - Dr. Ravi R. Paper presented at this National Conference on HSR. NIHFW, New Delhi, 14-18 Dec. 1992 Pg. 1-7.
9. Status of Health Systems Research (HSR) in India - Indira Murali Paper presented in National Conference on Health Systems Research, NIHFW, New Delhi, December 14-18, 1992 Pg. 1, 19-20, 25.
10. Concepts of Health Behaviour Research, SEARO Regional Health Papers No. 13, World Health Organisation, Regional Office for South East Asia, New Delhi, 1987 pg. 29-32.
11. The concept of Health Service Research SEARO Technical Publications 1 World Health Organisation, Regional Office for South East Asia, New Delhi, 1983 Pg. 6.

Chapter–27

India's Preparation for Disaster Reduction: An Overview

During the International Decade for Natural Disaster Reduction (IDNDR), the country will have to pay more attention towards public awareness and preparedness for the people living in known disaster-prone areas. Special training is required to medical, paramedical, voluntary workers in relief and rescue work.

Disaster by definition involves disruption of human ecology which cannot be absorbed by the adjustment capacity of the affected community within its own resources[1]. According to their genesis, disasters fall into two broad groups, viz (a) Natural disasters consequent to the fury of nature and (b) man made disasters which may be intentional or non-intentional (accidental)[2] .Although a determined human effort can totally, to a great extent prevent man-made disasters, the same does not hold good in respect of natural disasters which have a growing concern of mankind all over the world particularly during the last 3 decades or so. There is a growing awareness also that though it may not be possible to prevent natural disasters but these can be certainly tackled effectively through adequate preparedness to mitigate the loss of human life and property. It is against this background that on 11 Dec. 1989 the United Nations General Assembly proclaimed 1990's as the international Decade for Natural Disaster Reduction (IDNDR), beginning from Ist Jan. 1990, to initiate a concerted global effort to reduce the destruction impact of natural disasters which alone during the past two decades killed an estimared 3 million people.[3]

India is supposed to demarcate the disaster prone areas and work out the details of their increasing impact in terms of loss of life, physical damage and effect on economic developments. The country is supposed to apply the scientific and technological progress to disaster mitigation[4].

India's proneness to Natural Disasters

On the basis of grographic and climatic considerations, India can be divided into 5 zones acording to its disaster proneness to natural disaster as under.

1. **Northern Mountain Region including footnills:** This region is prone to strong snow storms leading to land slides and strong cold wave. Besides this, the entire Northern part from Hindukush to Eastern Himalayas, lies in earthquake prone belt of violent Subterranian volcanic activity.

2. **Indo-Gangetic Plain's:** Heavy rains during monsoon make these plains vulnerable to floods.

3. **Deccan Plateau:** A drought prone area.

4. **The Western Desert:** A drought prone area.

5. **Coastal Areas:** They are prone to sea erosion, cyclones and tidal waves.[4]

The disaster proneness varies widely form state to state. In 1990 alone, floods and cyclones claimed 1422 human lives in India; damaged about 2 million houses affecting 57.2 million people in 197 districts of 19 states/UTs: The crop area affected was 4.5 million hectares[5].

Some of the worst natural disasters in India in the recent past whose memory is still fresh in our minds, include (i) tropical cyclone on Andhra Pradesh Coast in 1977 which claimed more than 10,000 deaths and again an severe cyclone assuming devastation during 1989 (ii) Earthquake in Koyna Nagar:, Maharashtra (1967) Kinnaur and Lahaul Spiti in Himachal (1975), Bihar (1988), Garwhal Hills (1991) and Latur, Maharashtra (1993). The last one claimed a death toil of over 12,000 and many more were injured.

India is located in the South East Asia Region of WHO which ranked 4th amongst the most disaster prone regions in the world.

Progress in tackling Natural Disasters

The progess made in tackling disasters since India's independence reveals some important achievements:-

1. India became member of the World Meterological Organisation on 23 Mar, 1950.
2. Launching a National Flood Control Organisation in 1954.
3. Setting up of Brahmaputra Board in 1981.

The main activities since launching of National Flood Control Programme (1954) include-construction of embankments and drainage channels, town protection schemes, raising the level of flood prone villages, completion of reservoir projects, flood forecasting and warning for different river basins.

Indian Meterorological Dept. (IMD) also plays a key role in forewarning the disasters. It has 5 centers (Calcutta, Bhubaneshwar, Vishakahapatnam, Madras and Bombay) for detection and tracing of cyclones, storms and satellite imagery facillite and cyclone warning Radars provided to various cyclone warning centres. In addition, it has 31 Special Observation Posts set up along East Cost of India. For all ships, out at sea warning are issued 6 times a day.

Insat Disaster Warning System (DWS) recievers have been installed during the first phase of 100 stations, primarily in the coastal areas of Tamil Nadu and Andhra Pradesh. This has been proved highly reliable from of communicaton system for cyclonic warnings during Chirale cyclone (1989) and Machalipatnam cyclone in 1990[6] . The Snow and Avalanche Study Establishement (SASE) in Manali (H.P.) has been issuing warning to the people about avalanches 24 to 48 hours in advance.

For tracking any disaster every state has a full fledged Secretariat Wing under Relief Commissioner/Secretary for proper co-ordination at district level. In case of need, the state Governement can approach the Centre for help in repsect of finance, manpower, and material. At the Centre, the Ministry of Agriculture is the nodal ministry for co-ordination of all activities during any natural disaster. Since health is an important part of the disaster management, in the Directorate General of Health Services under Ministry of Health there is a Special Wing called the Emergency Medical Relief Wing which co-ordinates all activities relating to health. At the district level, the Collector forms a small commitee which assesses the degree of devastation and organises rescure and relief work and informs the State Govt. Relief Secretary/ Commissoner and works directly under Chief Secretary. The State Govt. officials/Ministers concerned visit the affected area to oversee relief operation and releases funds required later. The Central Teams including the members and officials from Health Ministry also visit the areas to assess the magnitude of the problems and recommed central assistance. The United Nations has a special body called UNDRO (Office of the United Nationas Disaster Relief Co-ordinator) which can always be approached for extra help whenever needed. The WHO and UNDP and other voluntary Organisation help in all major disasters.

Areas of Special Concern During IDNDR

During IDNDR, the country wil have to pay more atttention towards public awareness and preparedness in respect of people residing in known disaster prone areas. Special training is required to medical, paramedical, voluntary workers in relief and rescue work.

Refereness

1. Verma B.K. The Disaster Profile of India. Disaster Management (A. Report on Workshop held at Nagpur on 14-18 Oct. 1986, sponsored by the WHO) DGHS, Ministry of Health & FW, Ist Edn, 1987, pp. 8-19.

2. Urmil AC and Sandhu MS. Disasters- An Incresing Awareness, CHEB, Swasth Hind, Vol XXXV. No.7 Jul. 90 pp 160-162.

3. United Nations International Decade for National Disaster Reduction, CHEB Swasth Hind Vol XXV. No. 3-4 Mar-Apr 91. p. 80.

4. Mandal HS, Natural Disaster, Disaster Management (A Report DGHS, Ministry of Health & FW, Ist Edn, 1987 pp 30-33.

5. Pant MC Natrual Disaster Reduction Swasth Hind Vol XXXV, NO. 3-4 Mar-Apr 9, pp 65-69

6. Gopala Rao VV, India National Setellite (INSAT) Disaster Warning System. Swasth Hind vol XXXV, No. 3-4, Mar-Apr 91, pp 81-82.

Chapter–28

World Mental Health : Issues and Challenges

The four decades after the Second World War have seen vast economic, political and social changes worldwide and this, in turn, has led to tremendous improvement in health status of the world community. While physical health has improved world over, mental health status has remained stagnant or rather has deteriorated. Of late, increase in the incidence of clinical depression, schizophrenia, dementia and other forms of chronic mental illnesses have emerged as important health problems. Some of these illnesses are due to crushing psychic and social burden imposed by urbanisation and modernisation of rural cultures. The social, political and economic changes have been also accompanied by increase in the rate of alcoholism, drug abuse and suicide. Violence against women, children and the aged has become a common feature in most countries of the world.

Mental, behavioural and social health problems are increasing the health burden of the globe. According to a recent World Bank study, psychiatric diseases are the largest causes of lost years of quality of life. Hundreds of million of women, men and children suffer from mental illnesses while a large number experience distress from consequences of violence, dislocation, poverty and exploitation. Substance abuse and other behaviour related problems affect the lives of countless adolescents, young adults and the elderly.

The salient findings of the recent research studies have revealed the magnitude of the problem. Mental health problems alone make up 8.1 per cent of the global burden of disease. Of the disorders considered in the World Bank's estimates, depressive disorders, self inflicted injuries, Alzheimer's disease and other dementias and alcohol dependence cause the largest burden followed by epilepsy, psychosis, drug dependence and post traumatic stress disorder. It is projected that the total number of causes of schizophrenia in low income societies will increase from 11.7 million in 1985 to 24.4 million by 2000 AD - a 45% increase due to demographic changes. Mental retardation and epilepsy rates are 3-5 times higher in low income societies as compared to developed societies. Depressive and anxiety disorders together are responsible for 1/4th to 1/3rd of all primary health care visits worldwide. Distress from these disorders often go unrecognised. In selected Asian and African countries, upto 90 per cent of patients with epilepsy do not receive proper treatment. What is of more concern to us is that by the year 2025, three quarters of the elderly with dementia-roughly 80 million will live in low income countries. Similarly, at present an estimated 5-10 per cent of all persons in globe are affected by alcohol related diseases.

It is interesting to note that 85 per cent of 3 billion people afflicted by natural disasters between 1967 and 1991 live in Asia. About one third of disaster victims suffer from significant mental stress. Suicide is usually listed among top 10 causes of death in societies and among the top 2 or 3 causes for youth. The risk for suicide among those who abuse alcohol is 50-100 times greater than general population. Depression is also a frequent cause for suicide. An estimated 34 per cent of global burden of disease is due to behaviour related problems such as violence, diarrhoeal diseases, AIDS & STDs and other unintentional injuries. This means that more than one third of global burden of diseases could be prevented by changes in behaviour, better nutrition, immunisation, and reduction of violence. Rates of domestic violence against married women vary from 20-25 per cent. The rates are particularly high in association with alcohol abuse among men.

Quite simply, we are in the midst of a largely unheralded crisis in world mental health. Faced with a choice between reducing deficits and investing resources to address this mental health burden, poor and rich nations alike have opted to reduce deficits. Because many mental health problems such as substance abuse, violence, suicide and dementia are encountered in low income and high income societies alike. Solutions that work in one setting have potential applications in others. Contrary to prevailing beliefs, there are cost-effective treatments for certain psychiatric conditions e.g. depression, epilepsy and schizophrenia and some of others can be prevented. There are many promising local experiments and demonstration projects. In fact, there is much that low income countries can teach their wealthier neighbours if only information is shared. Even for these conditions for which treatment and prevention are at present available, there is enough knowledge to develop policies and programme and to generate research to obtain information crucial for the future. In spite of this, there is a worldwide failure to give priority to mental health problems. Mental health represents one of the last frontiers in the improvement of human conditions. In the face of widespread stigma and negligence, mental health must now be placed on the international agenda.

Recently, a collaborative research project was initiated comprising experts from more than 30 nations. It was probably the first systematic attempt to assess the burden of suffering imposed by mental, social and behavioural health problems with special reference to low income societies in Asia, Africa, Latin America and the Middle East. The World Mental Health Report published in May, 1995 are couple of years intensive study by experts of various countries and researchers in the Department of Social Medicine at Harvard Medical School, warned about the emergence of a crisis in world mental health. This study highlighted the growing burden of mental, behavioural, social problems in third world countries, examined the sources of substantial morbidity rates and their relation to development, and also assessed current efforts to cope with them. The study identified opportunities for effective mental health interventions, method of treatment, culturally appropriate preventive programmes and sound policy formation. It relates to mental health consequences of violence, dislocation, poverty and the disenfranchisement of women to the most pressing economic, political and environmental problems of our time. Brief description of the key findings and recommendations for policy of research innovations have been incorporated in this report.

If we are to improve the state of mental health, there must be an international comparison to accord priority to mental health policies and programmes so that mental health problems are viewed by the international community as what they are — a great threat to political and economical stability of the world. In addition to UN as a whole, the campaign must involve WHO, UN High Commission for Refugees, UNDP, UNICEF, the World Bank, NGOs, regional and national agencies, as well as the media, business, educational networks, health professions and networks of health and policy professionals.

It is felt that such a commitment from United Nations is needed to focus world attention on this most pressing, yet least immediately visible of health problems. It is simply unacceptable that in the closing days of the 20th century in so many countries the chronically mentall ill patients are still abandoned in conditions of filth and brutality without treatment or rehabilitation to the detriment of their human rights and dignity.

But no call for action, no matter how scientifically planned, can accomplish anything if world turns a deaf ear to it. Thus first and most important recommendation is that the UN should soon declare a year of mental health and the year 1996-2006 to be designated as WHO Decade of Mental Health.

References

1. World Mental Health : Problems and Priorities in Low Income Countries—Robert Desjarlais, Leon Essenberg, Byrou Good & Arthur Vleinman, Oxford Unibversity Press, 1995.

2. Mental Health Care in India and the Global Context — Ravi Kapur. A paper presented in World Mental Health Conference hosted by Rajiv Gandhi Institute of Contemporary Studies, New Delhi 6-8 April, 1995.
3. Alcohol Behaviour in a Socio Cultural Perspective - Davinder Mohan.
4. Mental Health I; Health for Millions July-August, 1994, Vol. 20 No. 4.

Index

U

V

W

Y

PUBLIC HEALTH AND SOCIAL ASPECTS

PUBLIC HEALTH AND SOCIAL ASPECTS

By

PROF. (COL.) P.K. DUTTA

KHAMA PUBLISHERS
NEW DELHI

PUBLIC HEALTH AND SOCIAL ASPECTS

First Published in India 1998

ISBN 81-85495-48-3

Published by:
A. Banerjee
for Khama Publishers
1770, Khawaspura, Pataudi House
Daryaganj, New Delhi-110002

Laser typeset at:
Printline
12-H, New Daryaganj Road,
New Delhi-110002

Printed at:
Super Printers
1893, Gali Behrem Beg,
Lal Kuan, Delhi

Dedicated
To
My Parents

Contents

SECTION IV
HEALTH EDUCATION

SECTION V
MISCELLANEOUS

Preface

Most of today's health problems are attributed to biological, social, environmental and individual factors for causation of illness and also for the subsequent progress in natural history of the disease. There is no denial of the fact that the social environment is very important in relation to health and disease of the human population.

With growing industrialisation, urbanisation and control of communicable diseases specially of parasitic and bacterial origin, there is emergence of non-communicable disease. In today's world, effects of social environment has distinct impact on the morbidity pattern specially in rural areas and urban slums. Many of the important public health problems are also related to life styles of people belonging to different strata of the societies and examples are many – Diabetes, obesity, coronary heart disease, Alcohal and drug abuses. The changes in value system also are reflected in an increasing trend of diseases associated with modern world.

The effects of social environemnt reflect on the complex of psycho social aspects influencing health and disease of the individauls, the communities and the nations. The social environment is unique to man and include cultural values, customs, habits, attitudes, beliefs, education, income, occupation, standard of community life and impact of social and political organisations. Hence it is essential to have proper understanding of social sciencces in general and sociology and cultural antropology in particular in order to appreciate impact of social environment and it's adverse effects on health and diseases. Sociology is the behaviour of man in society. The man's behaviour is affected not only by biological and physical environemnt, but also by social environment.

It is now being gradually realised by researchers and scientists from various disciplines that a number of factors are associated with health and disease. Some of the behavioural sciences including sociology, anthropology and psychology are closely interrelated with natural history of many diseases - right from etiology, diagnosis, preventive measures and rehabilitation. A holistic and interdisciplinary approach, therefore, is essential for research workers drawn from different disciplines including health and social sciences. Not many social scientists and public health specialists either singularly or jointly have indertaken relevant research studies to corelate social aspects of disease and health. The author had conducted a number of studies during the last 3 decades of his professional career including knowledge, application and practice (KAP) studies in the fields of communicable disease, family planning and MCH care.

The author has experienced during 25 years in medical teaching and research, that not many empirical studies/relevant literature on the subject could be cited for training post graduate students in medicine. Even for undergraduate students, this is a definite 'felt need' of psycho-social studies in health and disease, which could be a source of inspiration for medical sociologists. The community based social sciences research in the field of community medicine is very few and far between. Keeping this in mind, the author decided to compile the relevant articles/studies that were undertaken either by him, his colleagues and post-graudate students, during his 5 years tenure at AFMC, Pune and subsequently.

The importance of health education has been realised immensely during last few years so much so that it has been recognised as a speciality. Few national institutions like All India Institute of Hygiene and Public Health, Calcutta, Central Health Education Bureau, New Delhi, Gandhigram Inst. of Rural Development, Madurai, had been conducting Post Gradurate Diploma courses on the subject i.e., Diploma in Health Education. The reason for attaching so much imporatnce to the subject was because educators/planners realised that utilisation of health care delivery system etc.

after claborate planning, flop or remain fully under utilised because of lack of awareness among the beneficiaries. Hence it has been realised that clientele, for whom the health programme is meant, have to be properly educated and motivated, before rich dividends can be accrued. International Health agencies like WHO, UNICEF have been laying emphasis on the community participation and their full involment if we want to ensure optimal utilisation and active participation by the community. After gathering details on the health programme and after fully motivated only full participation by the community can be ensured.

This book is collection of 28 such articles which is divided into 6 sections.

Seciton 1 deals with medio social aspects of few communicable diseases, namely diarrhoeal diseases, sexually transmitted diseases, Measles and Smallpox. In this section, certain customs and beliefs among the study subjects about small pox and measles have also been studied.

Section 2 dealing with blindness has focussed on medicosocal and psychosocial profile of blind inmates of few homes.

Section 3 has highlighted about the medicosocial study of Menstrual Regulators (MR) & Medical Termination of Pregnancy (MTP) acceptors and also demographic profile of tubectomy acceptors.

Utilisation of health services by high risk children and of 'high risk' pregnant mothers have been brought out in Section 4 thus depicting causes of underutilisation of these essential services in slum areas.

In Section 4 a few articles on health education have been incorporated. These have been presented in a wider canvas and articles include smoking and its hazards, medicosocial problems of today's youth, geriatric population and their various problems, anaemia in pregnancy and cancer cervix, considered as scourge of women. This chapter also addresses other health and social issues like psychosocial aspects of hearing loss, diarrhoeal diseases under 5 children, population explosion and menace of intestinal helminthiasis.

Last chapter (Section 5) deals with a variety of other interesting topics life medicosocial study of paraplegics; tobacco smoking habits of army personnel, psychosocial profile of orphans, women to women education in devivery of non-formal health care, scope of Health System Research (HSR) in CSSM programme, India's preparation for disaster reduction and World Mental Health : Issues and Challenges.

In this book, an attempt has been made to present and analyse some of medicosocial and psychosocial issues related to health and disease.

The persons who initiated me in studying and writing articles on attitudes and beliefs about smallpox is none less than my revered teacher, Late Dr J. E. Park who has been one of the stalwarts in the field of community medicine. While I was enrolled as a postgraduate student in mid sixties under him, Dr. Park advised me to also initiate a research project on anthropological aspects of smallpox though my main topic of MD thesis was Evaluation of National Smallpox Eradication Pragramme in Gwalior District. The first article of my professional career on attitude and beliefs about smallpox was published in Armed Forces Medical Journal about 3 decades ago. Later on, I was granted 2 years study leave in late seventies and then I had the previlege of working with Prof. D. Banerjee at Jawaharlal Nehru Univeristy. He is also well known for his knowledge and command in the field of medical sociology and that too for his original and pioneering reserch. While working under him, I have also learnt a lot of various aspects of social sciences which could be applied in the field of social medicine. Both, Late Dr. J. Park and Dr. D. Banerjee my revered teachers inspired me to work in this field.

As mentioned earlier, very few studies have been conducted specially by the medical scientists in social aspects of health and disease. During the last two decades or so, though, few social scientists like Dr. K. Hasan, Dr. Sahu, Dr. Banerjee, etc. had undertaken a number of research studies which were mainly community based but hardly any medical scientists tried to initiate such projects. Even on review of literature, it was found that very few books/articles were available on this aspect. While teaching the undergraduate and postgraduate students at AFMC, Pune and most of the studies incorporated in the present publication is outcome of their research projects aundertaken by faculty members or postgraduate students. Few of my collegues were also keen to undertake projects on social aspects of health and were mostly community based projects. Prof. (Col.) A.C. Urmil, Dr. S.S. Ganguly and Late Col. (Dr.) T.K.G. Choudhary, my close friends and colleagues also had undertaken a number of studies based on social sciences. Other academic collegues and most of whom were postgraduate students during my tenure at AFMC whose names are worth mentiioning in bringing out the studies are Late Lt. Cols M. Kulkarni, Leo Vaz, Goutam Ghose, K.K. Sharma, P.K. Singh, Bhushan Kumar and S.K. Agarwal. All these colleagues from Army Medical Corps had been either jointly or singly working on various medico social aspects of health and disease. Col (Retd) Gopinathan, Prof. P.K. Somaya of, Karad Institute of Medical Sciences, Maharastra and Col. A.C. Urmil had always encourging me to take-up suitable research projects to correlate social sciences in health field. Inadvertantly, if any of my colleague's name has not been included, I owe an apology to them.

I would like to take this opportunity to thank Mr. Anupam Benerjee of Khama Publishers, Ansari Road, New Delhi and printers for bringing out the book in record time.

My thanks are also due to my wife Dr. (Mrs.) Mahuya Dutta and my children Pratik and Amrita for bearing with me while preparing the manuscript of the publication.